LITTLE MAN,
Wash Your
HANDS!

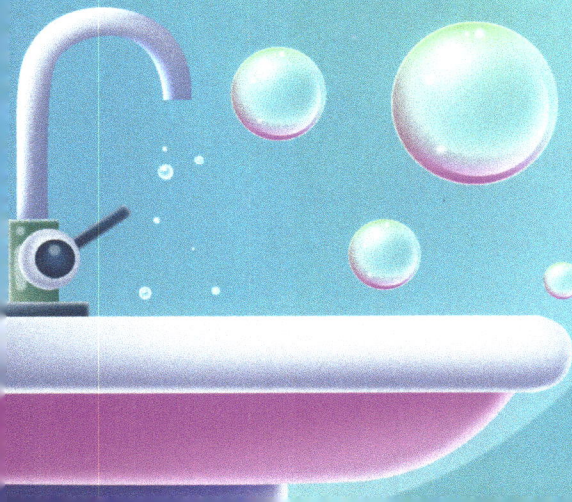

Dedication

This book is dedicated to all the littles I have ever taught. To all the OR staff who have heard me say "Gel in and Gel out" and know the art of hand washing is the first line of defense against surgical site infections. To my own littles, I love you.

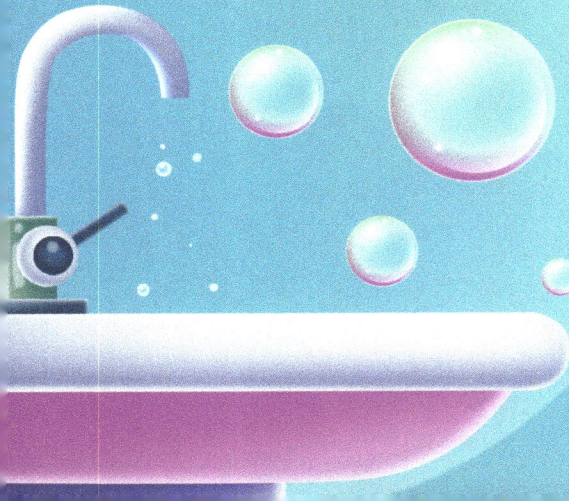

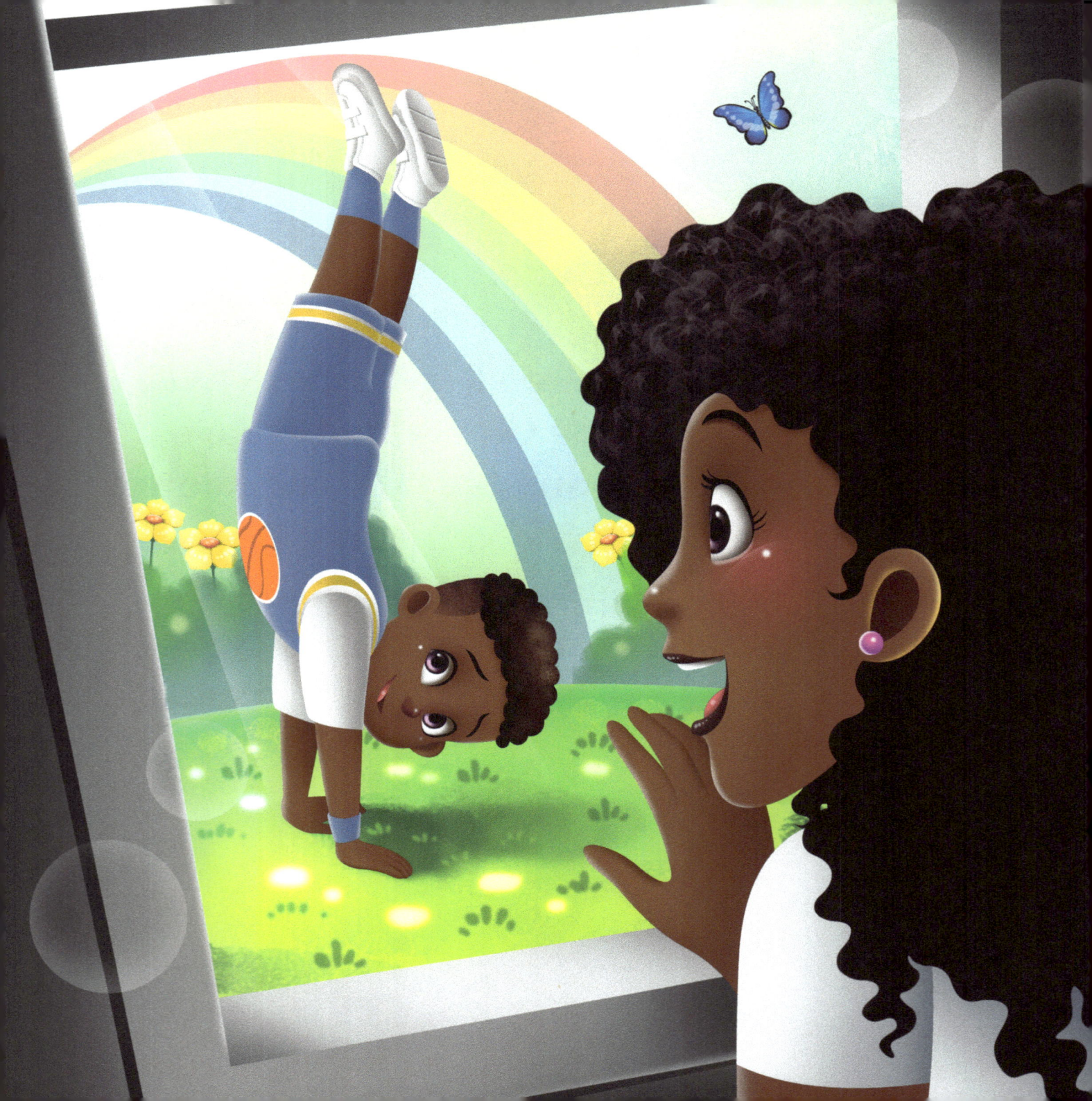

Little Man it is time to eat!
You better move those feet!

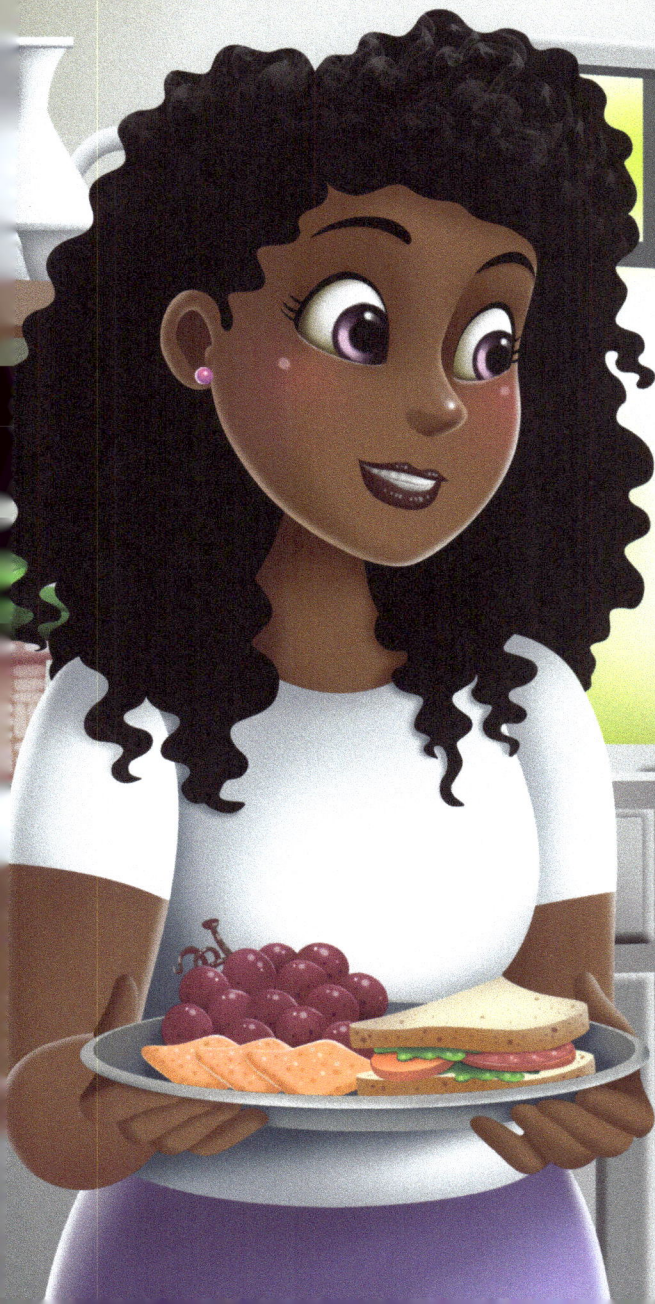

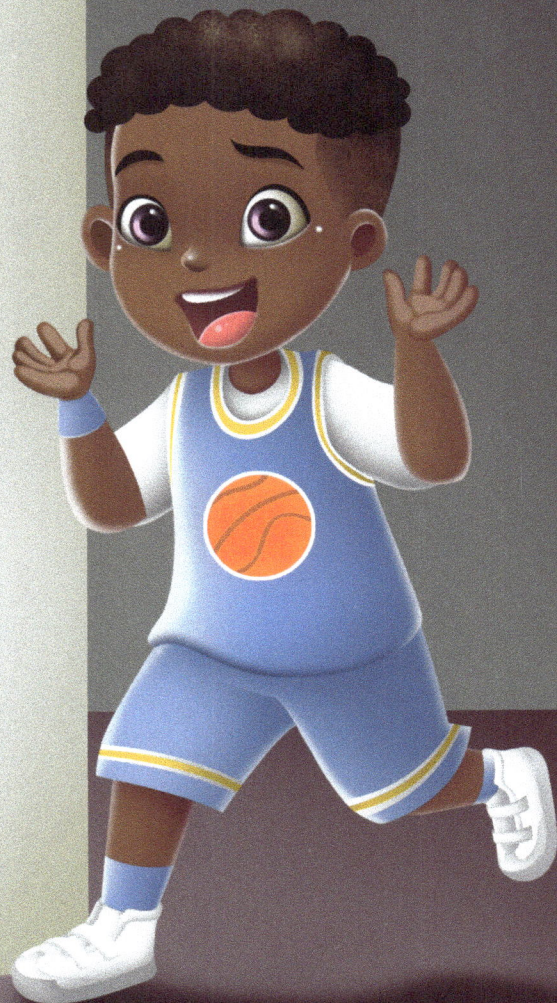

Hey, Little Man come give me a kiss
But do not touch this and this and this.
Be on the way to wash those hands,
No arguing with me, the order stands.

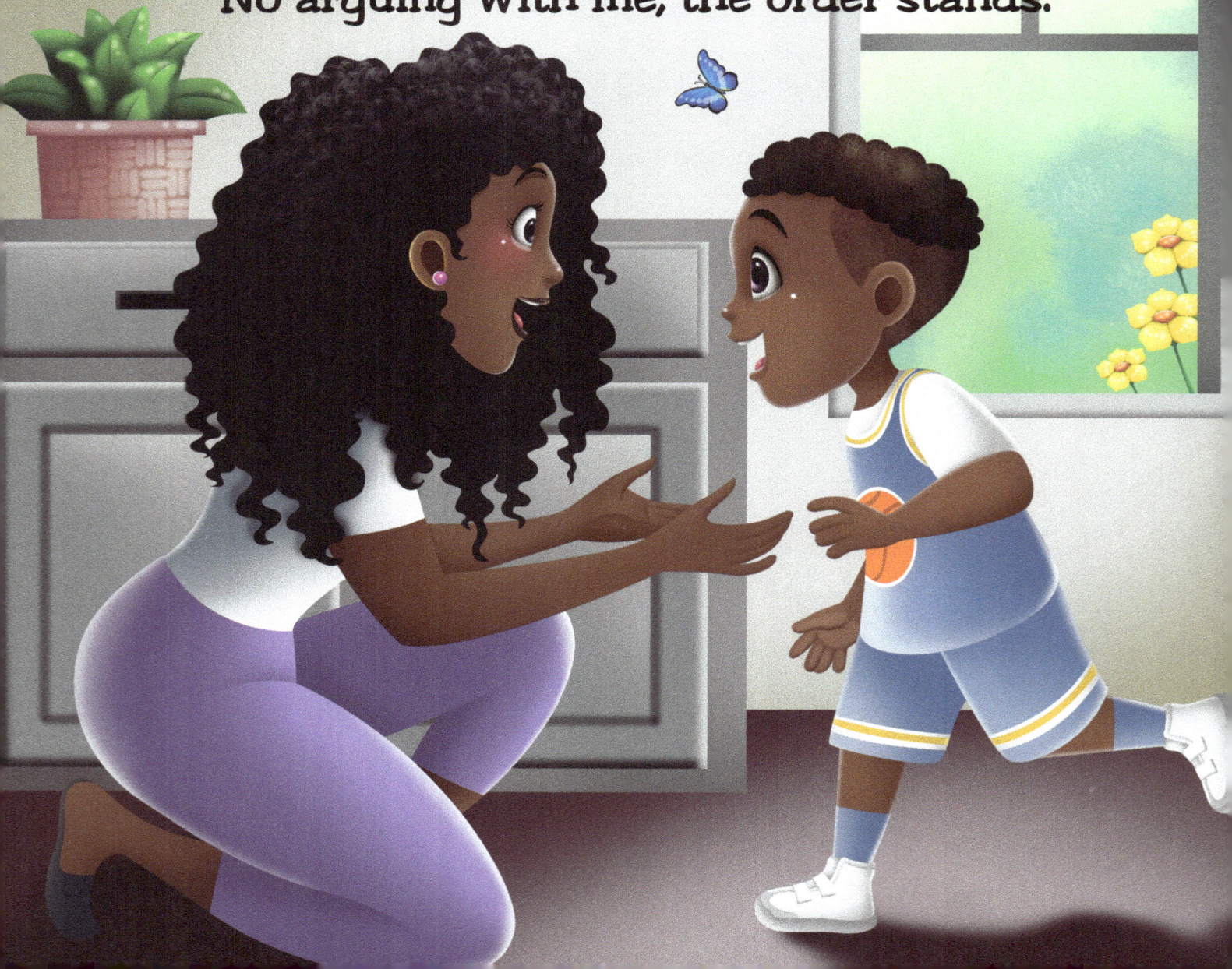

Not sure why, I was just playing outside.
But I do as I am told
So, I do not get a scold.

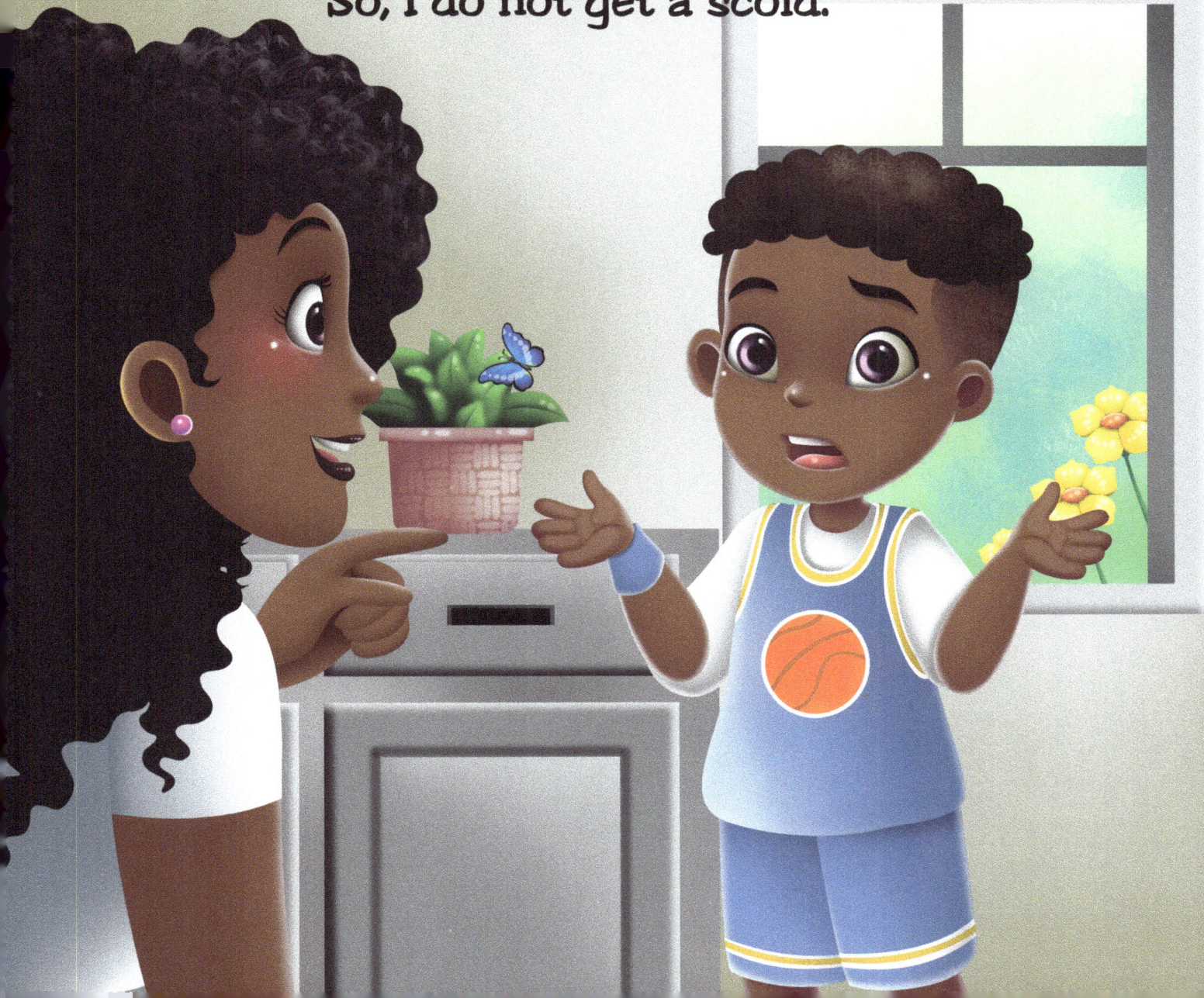

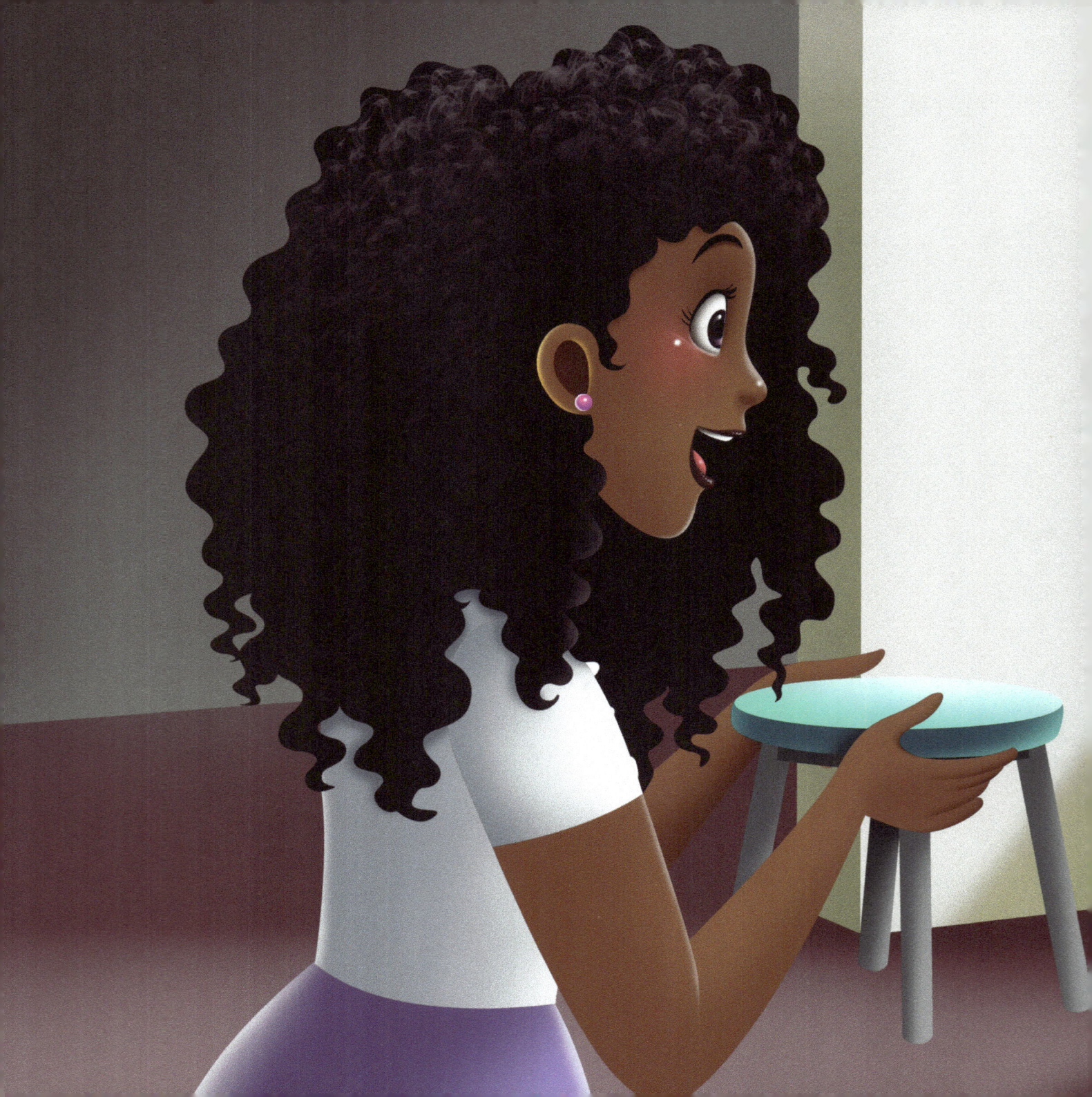

I run to the kitchen sink, but cannot reach.
So, Mama brings a stool to be a peach.
"Hey, Little Man! Do I need to help you with
this?" "I think I got this," as I pretend to
grab soap from the dish.

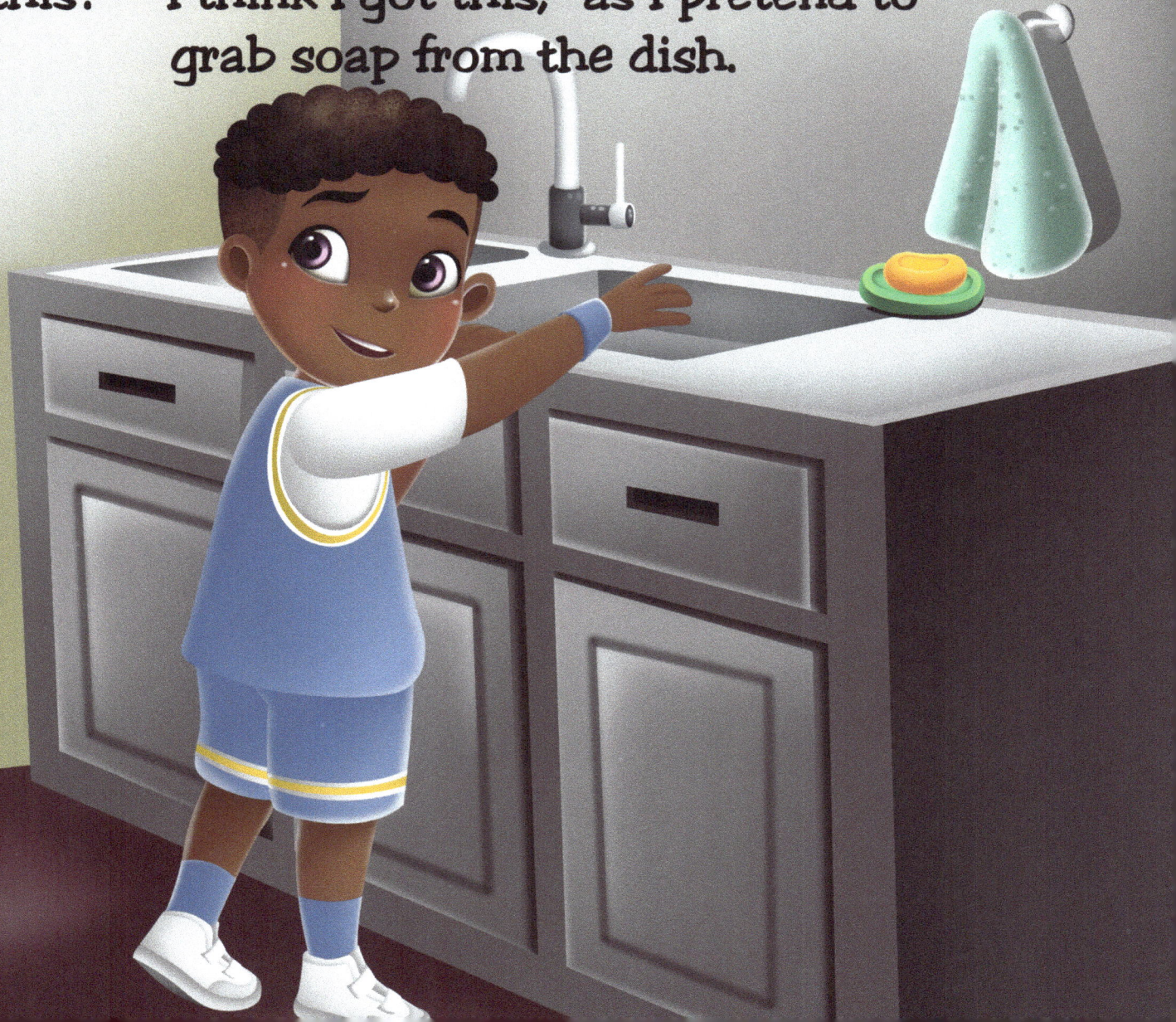

Mama spies my trick and gives me the eye,
I smile back at Mama just as sweet as pie.
Soap is what I know I need,
But I really just want to eat some beans.

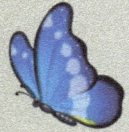

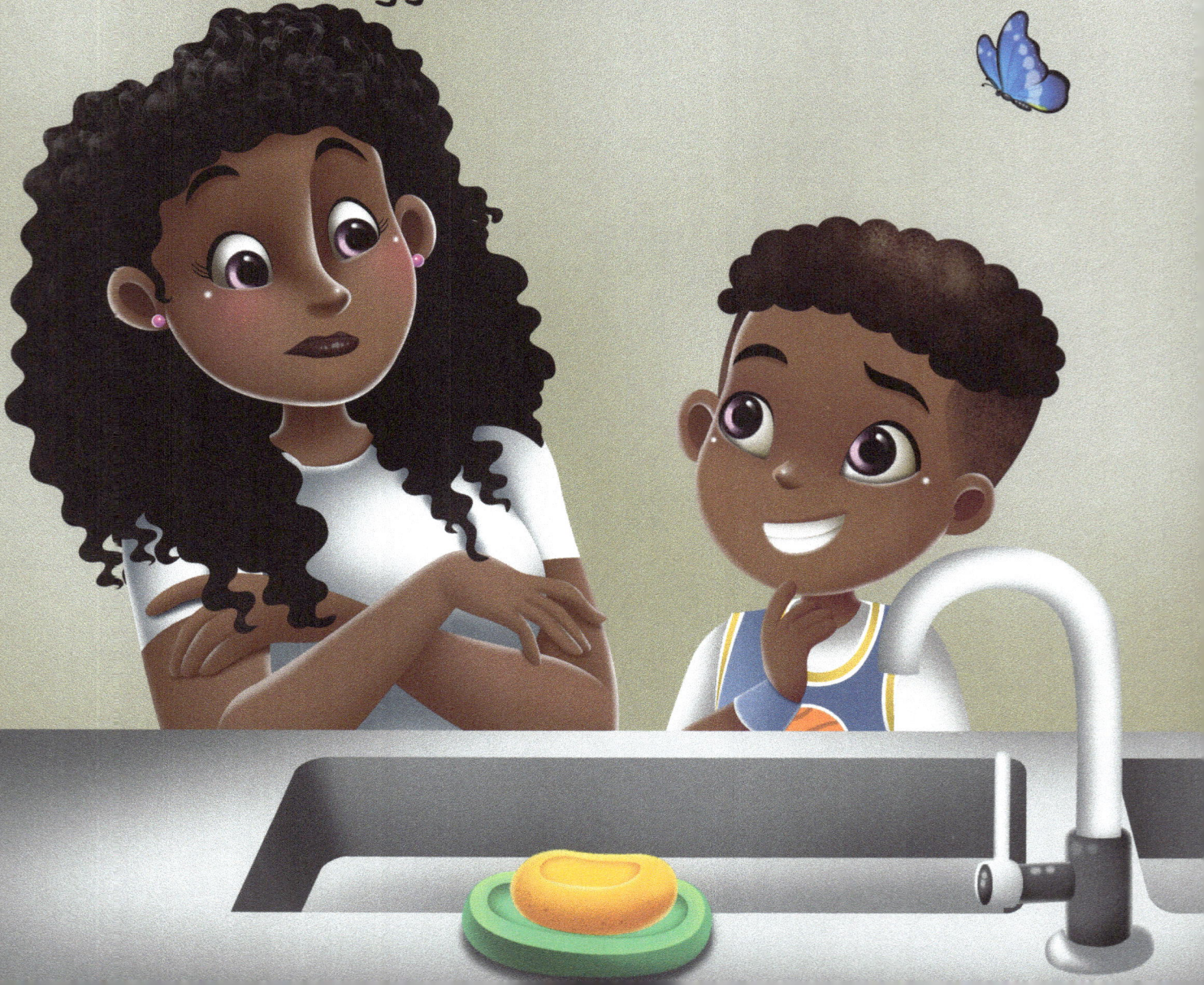

Little Man, I think you missed the soap.
I grab the soap, wash my palms, and hope.
I count ONE, TWO, THREE.
I am done and run the water until
the soap is all free.

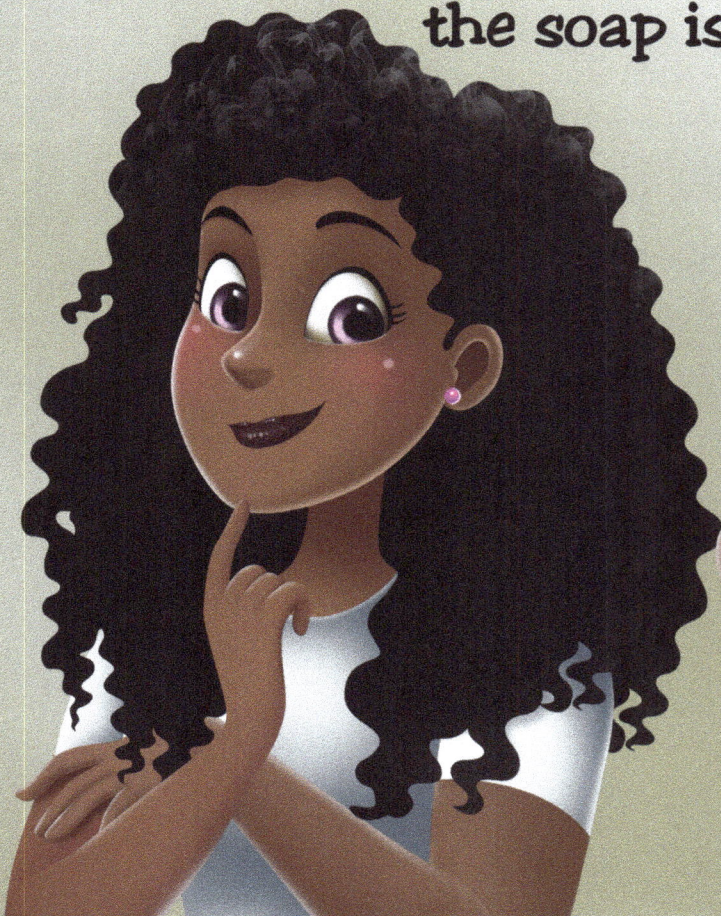

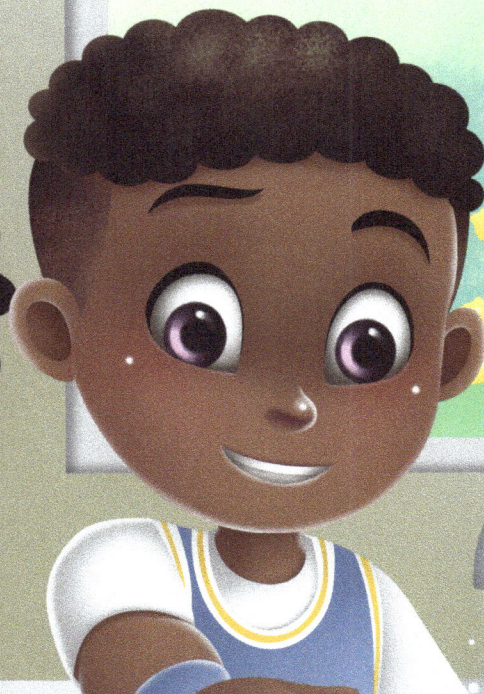

Hey, Little Man you forgot to wash your fingers,
Are you sure you don't want me to linger?
I can help you properly wash those hands,
So you are clean and germ free from all
those hand stands.

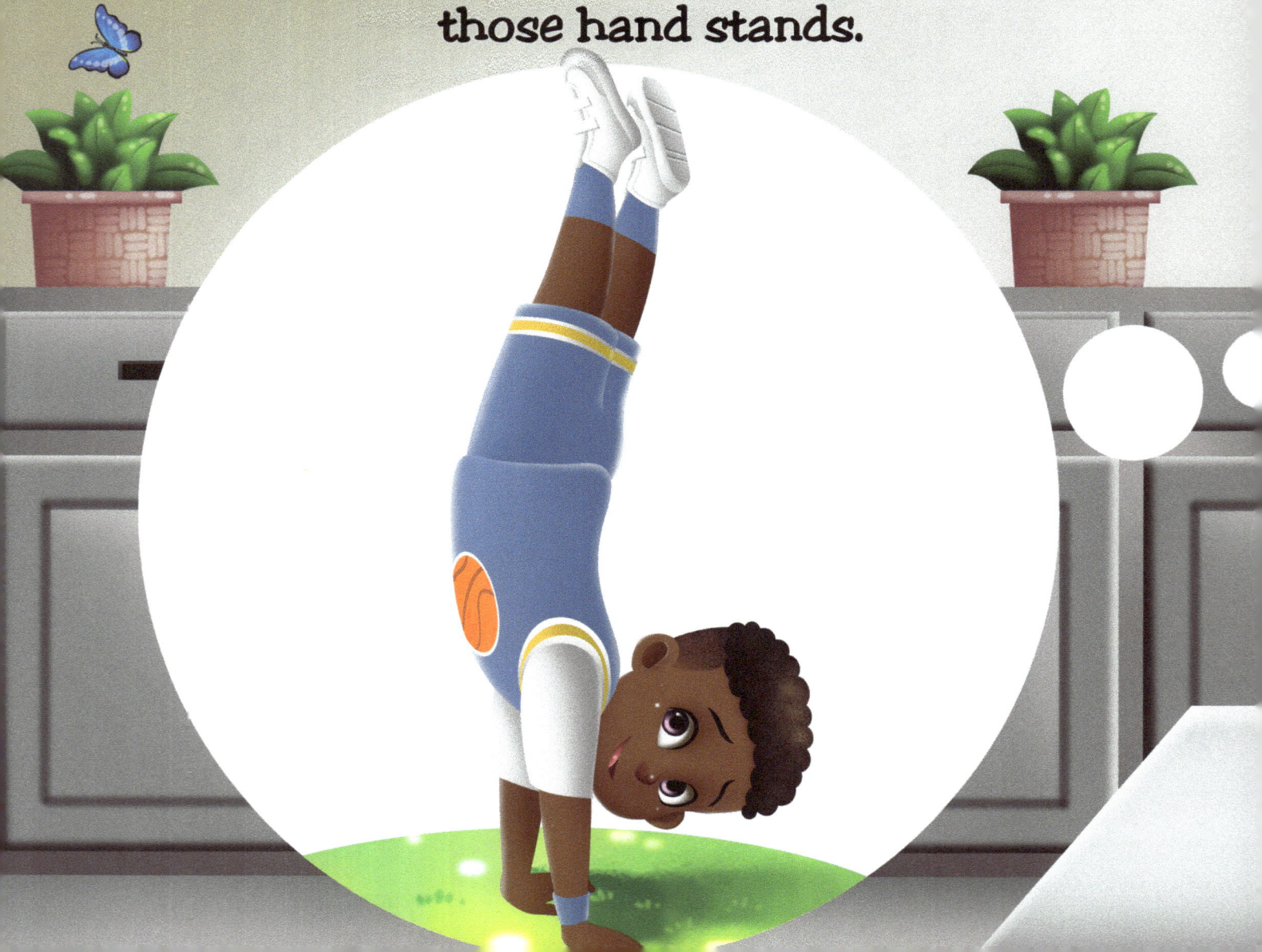

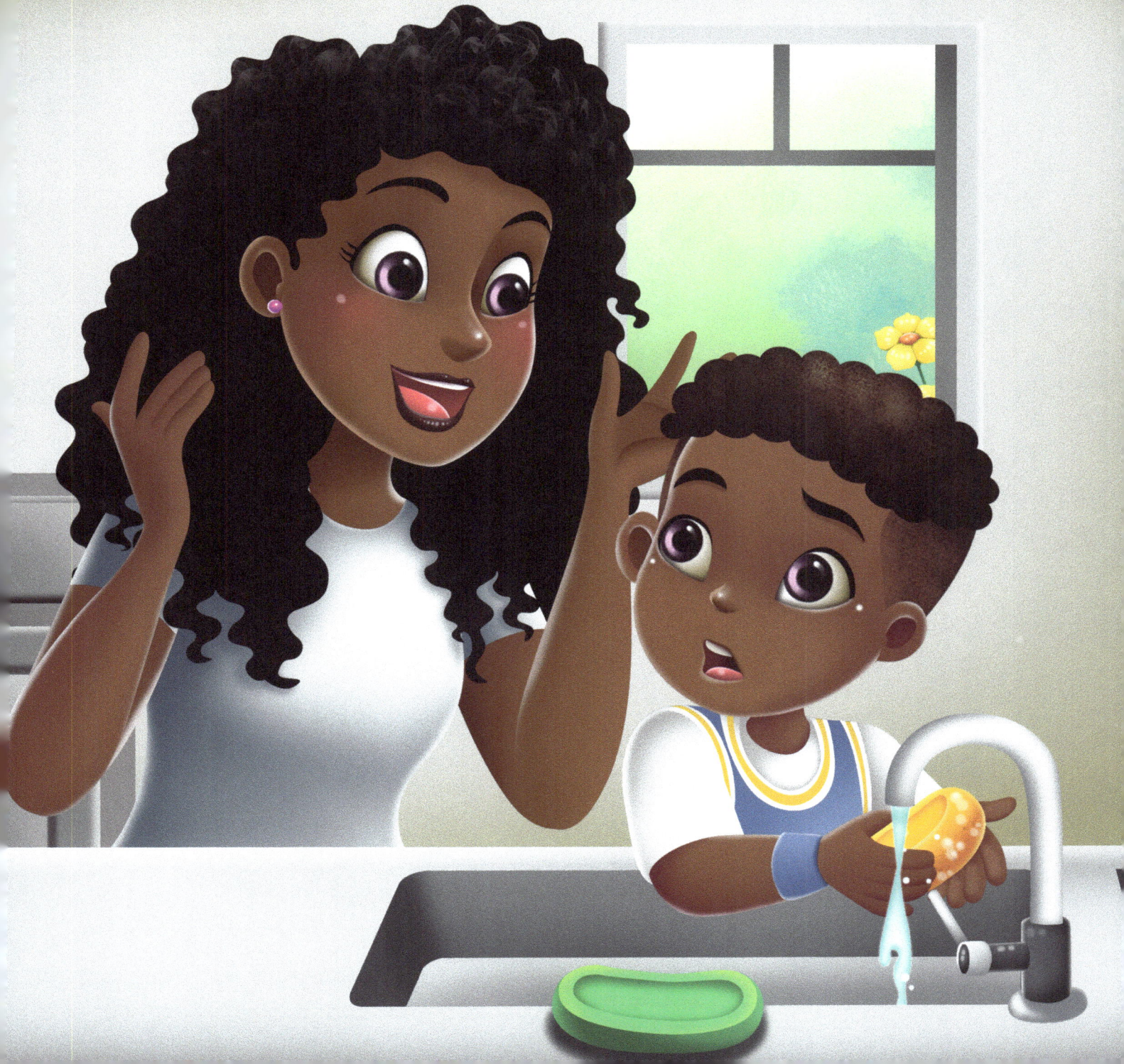

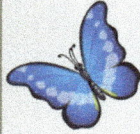

Ok Mama can you help me with this? This time, Mama gets her wish, As I ask for her help with this.

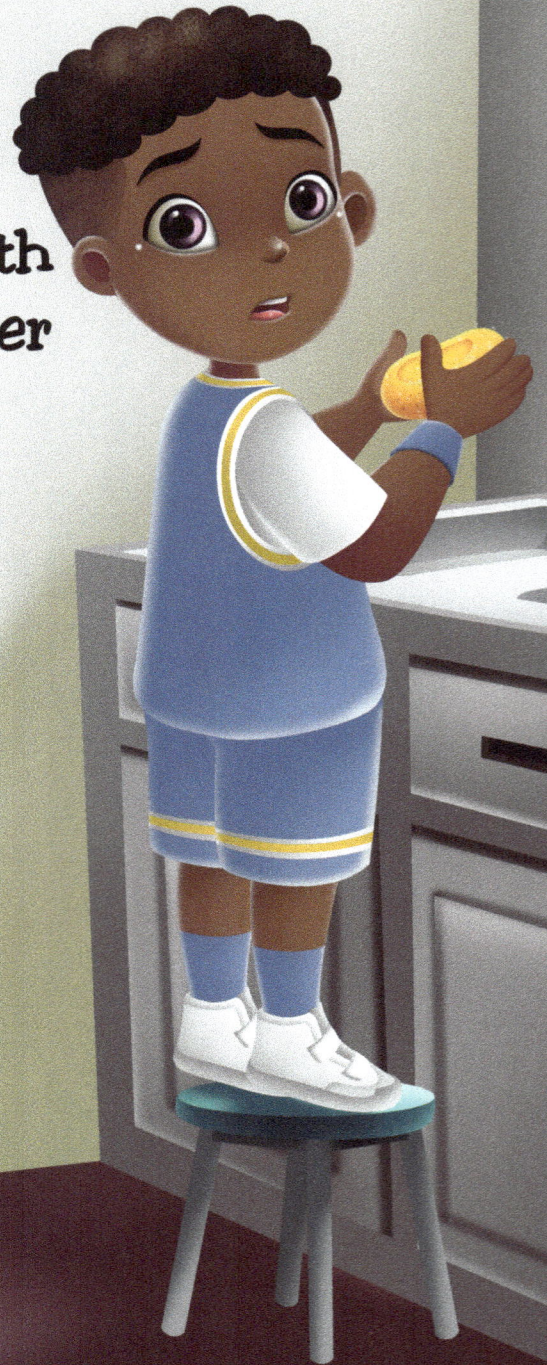

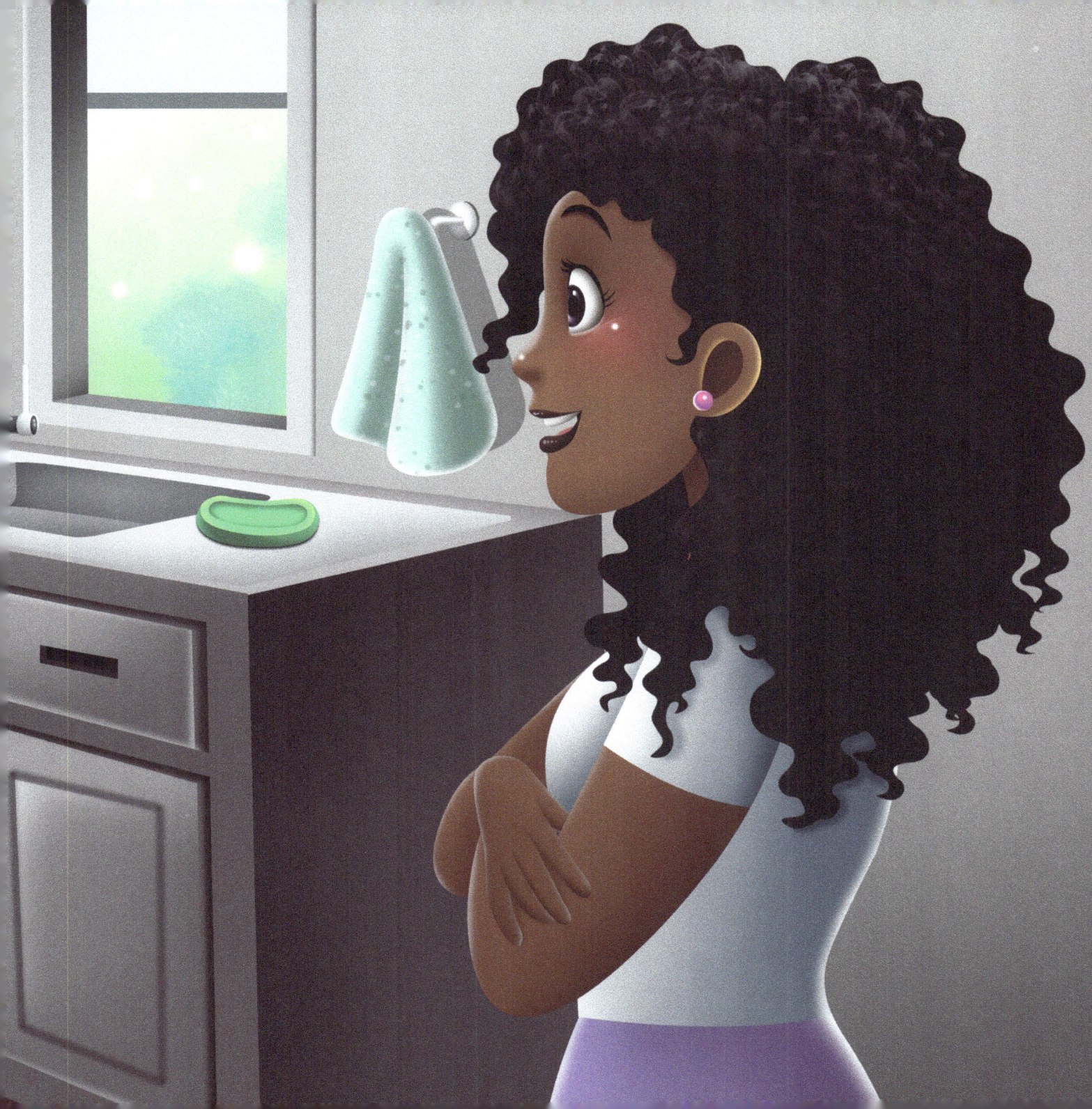

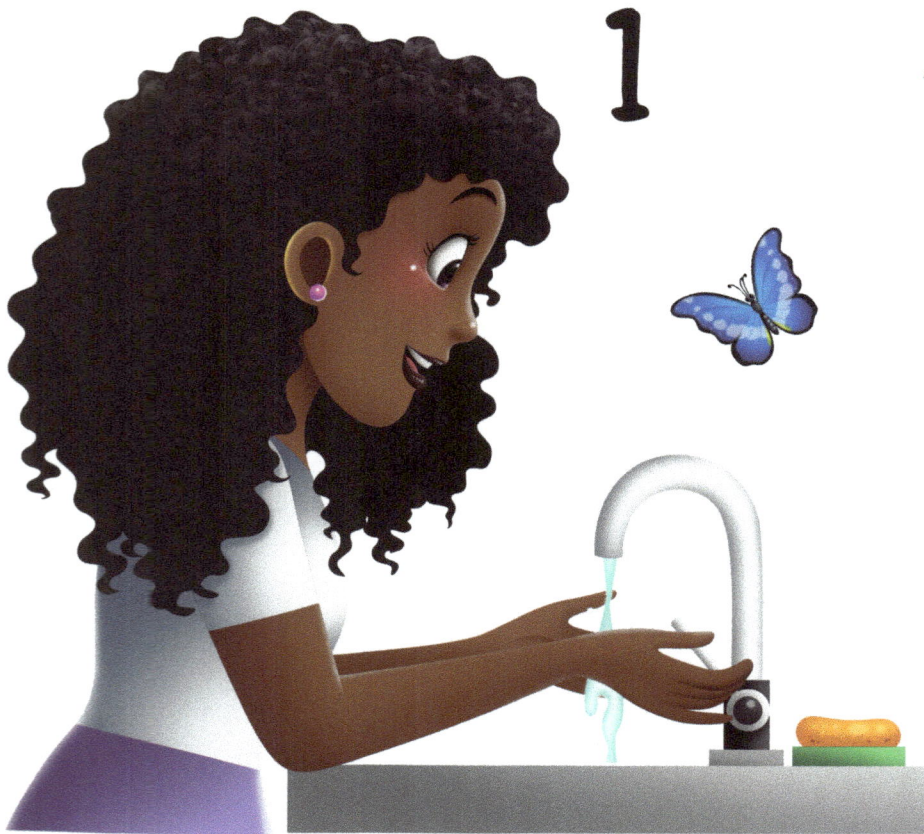

1

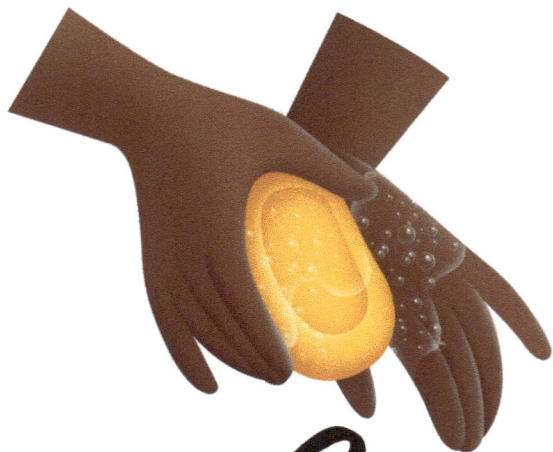

2

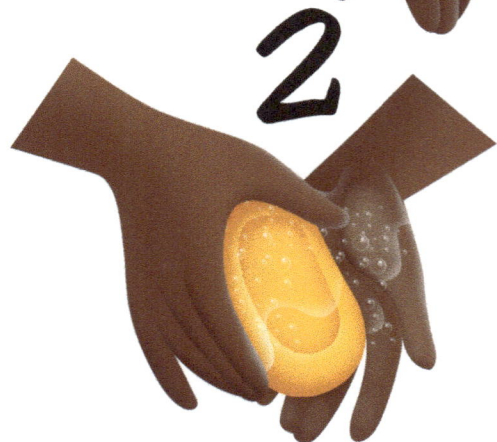

3

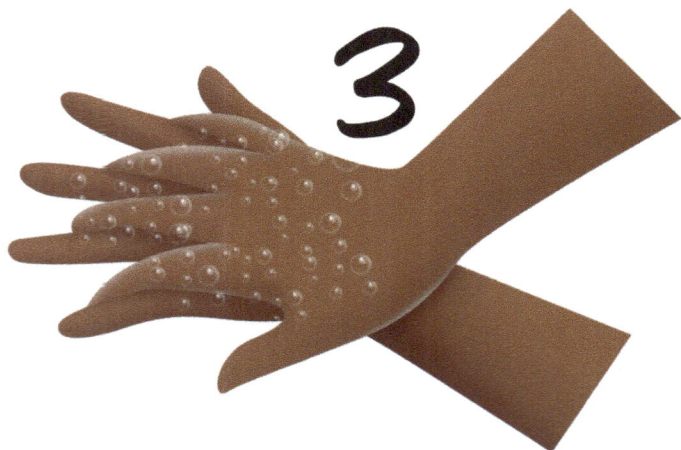

4

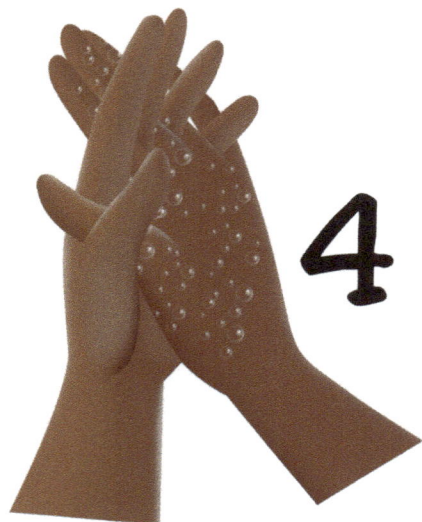

Yes, my love, washing your hands is even more important right now. Let me stand next to you and show you how:

Step 1: Get your singing voice warmed up "La, La, La."

Step 2: Turn the water on, rinse your hands, and start singing the Happy Birthday song.

Step 3: Rub soap on the front and back of your hands and keep singing your song.

Step 4: Wash in between and all around each of your 10 fingers—start with your thumb.

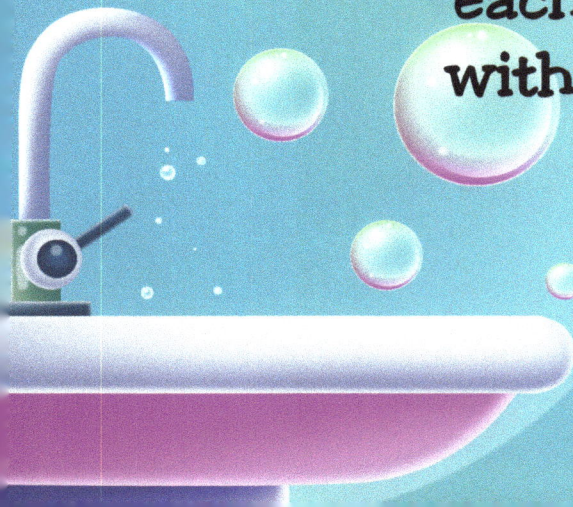

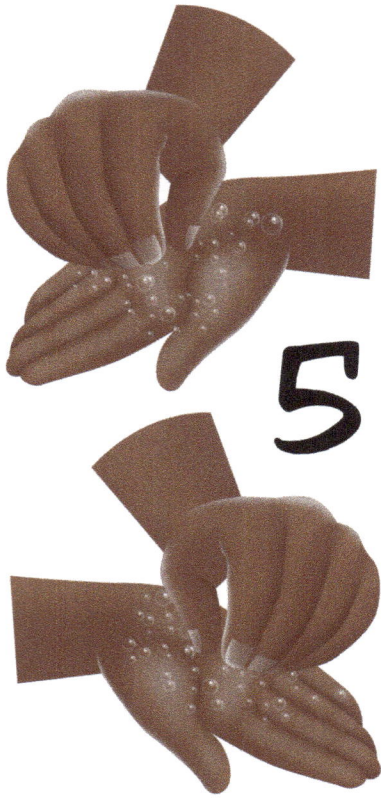

5

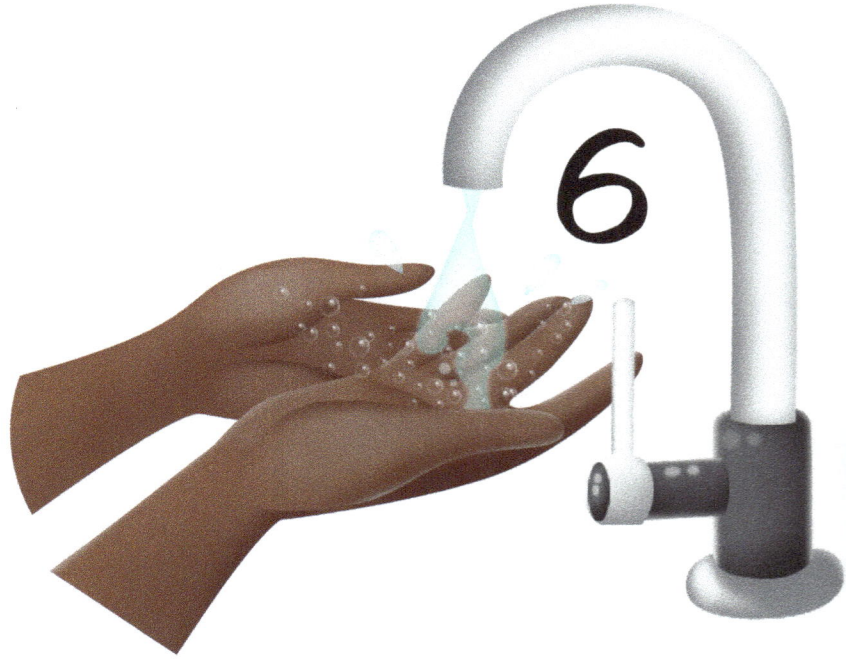

6

7

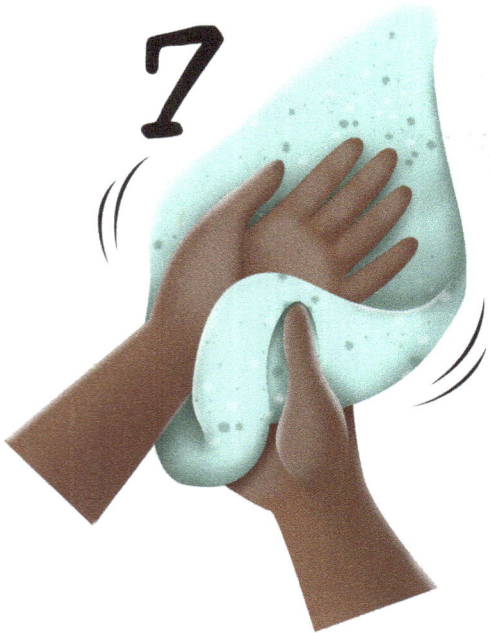

8

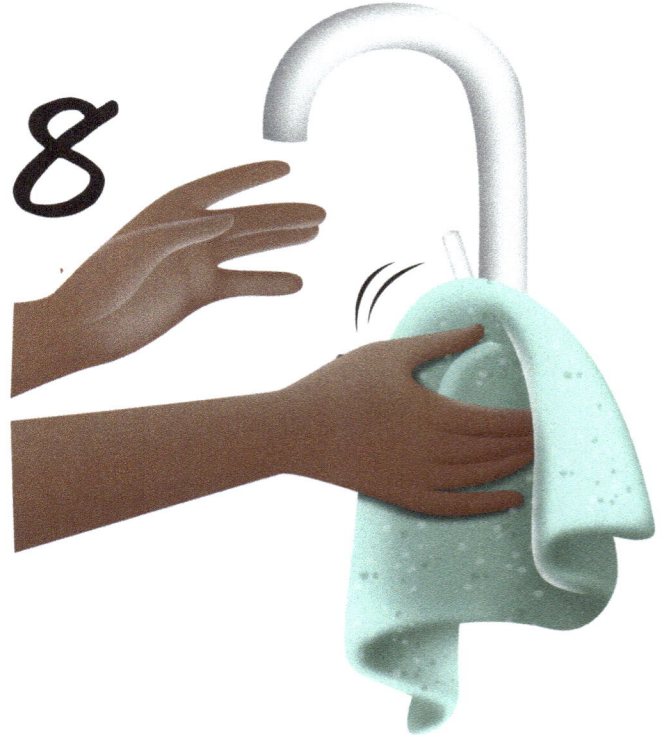

Step 5: Be sure to get underneath your fingernails while finishing up your song.

Step 6: Rinse all the soap off your hands with water.

Step 7: Dry your hands with a towel.

Step 8: Use that towel to turn off the faucet.

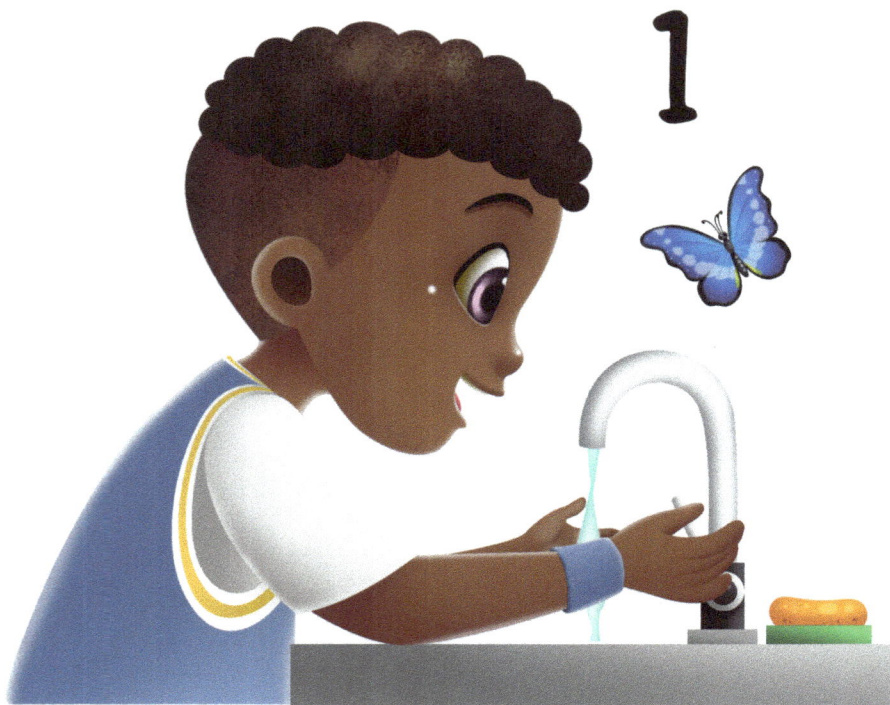
1

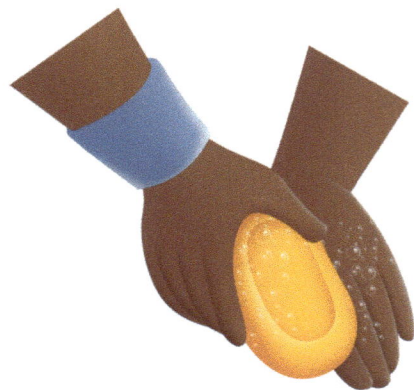
2

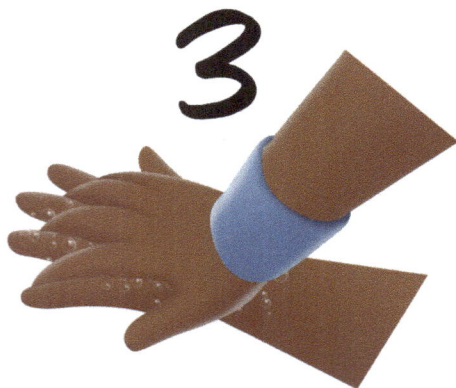
3

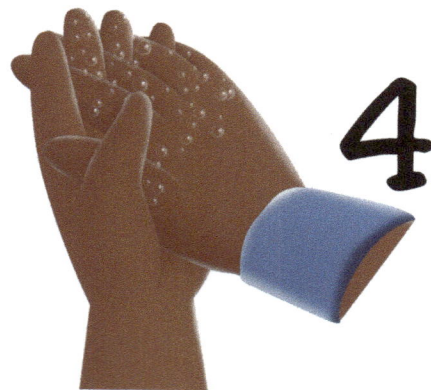
4

Once Mama shows me how,
I am ready to try it on my own right
now! I warm up my singing voice and jump
right into step 2:
Step 2: Turn the water on, rinse your
                hands, and start singing the
                Happy Birthday song.
Step 3: Rub soap on the front and back
                of your hands and keep singing
                your song.
Step 4: Wash in between and all around
                each of your 10 fingers—start
                with your thumb.

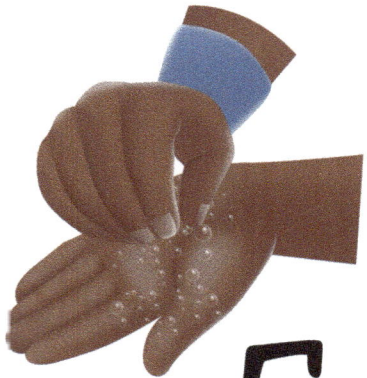

5

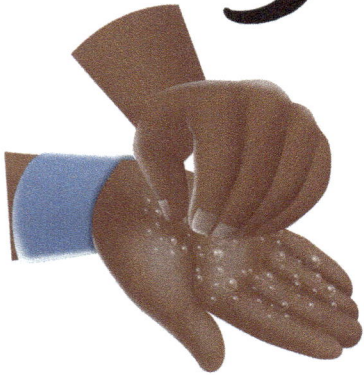

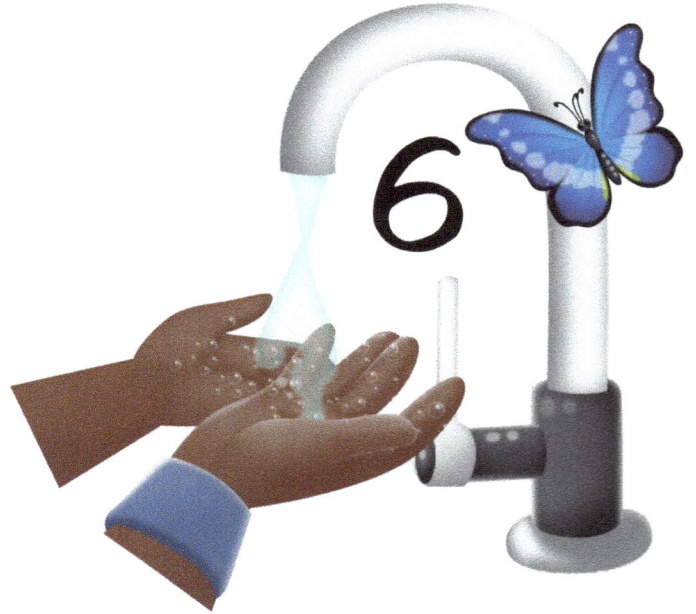

6

7

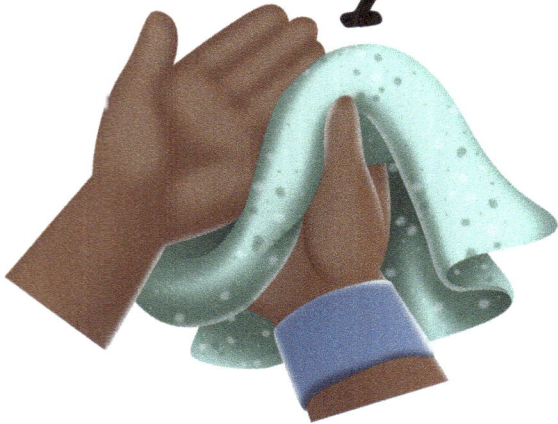

8

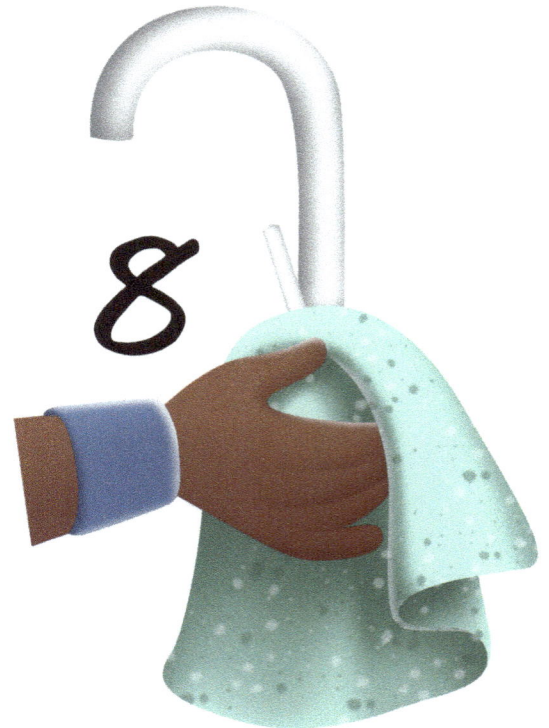

Step 5: Be sure to get underneath your fingernails while finishing up your song.

Step 6: Rinse all the soap off your hands with water.

Step 7: Dry your hands with a towel.

Step 8: Use that towel to turn off the faucet.

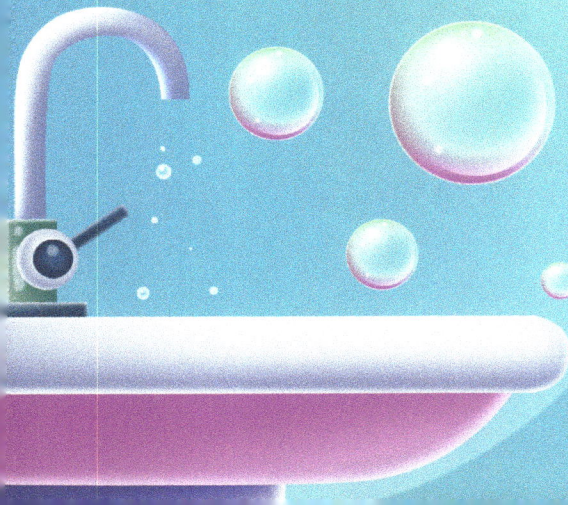

The next day at school we learn from operating room nurse, Mrs. Tish, That washing our hands to stop spreading germs is her wish. We can stop people from getting sick, If you wash those hands really quick.

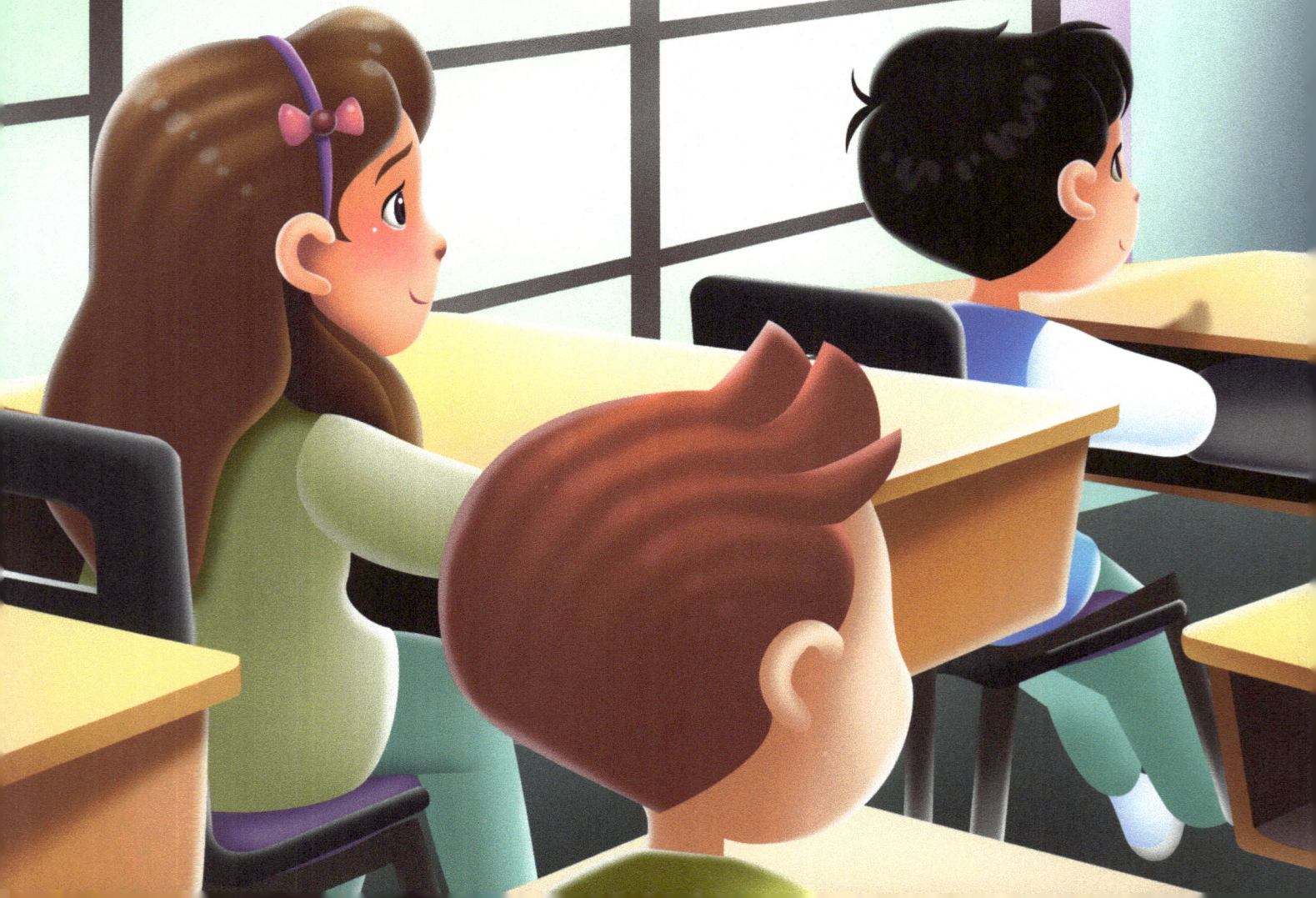

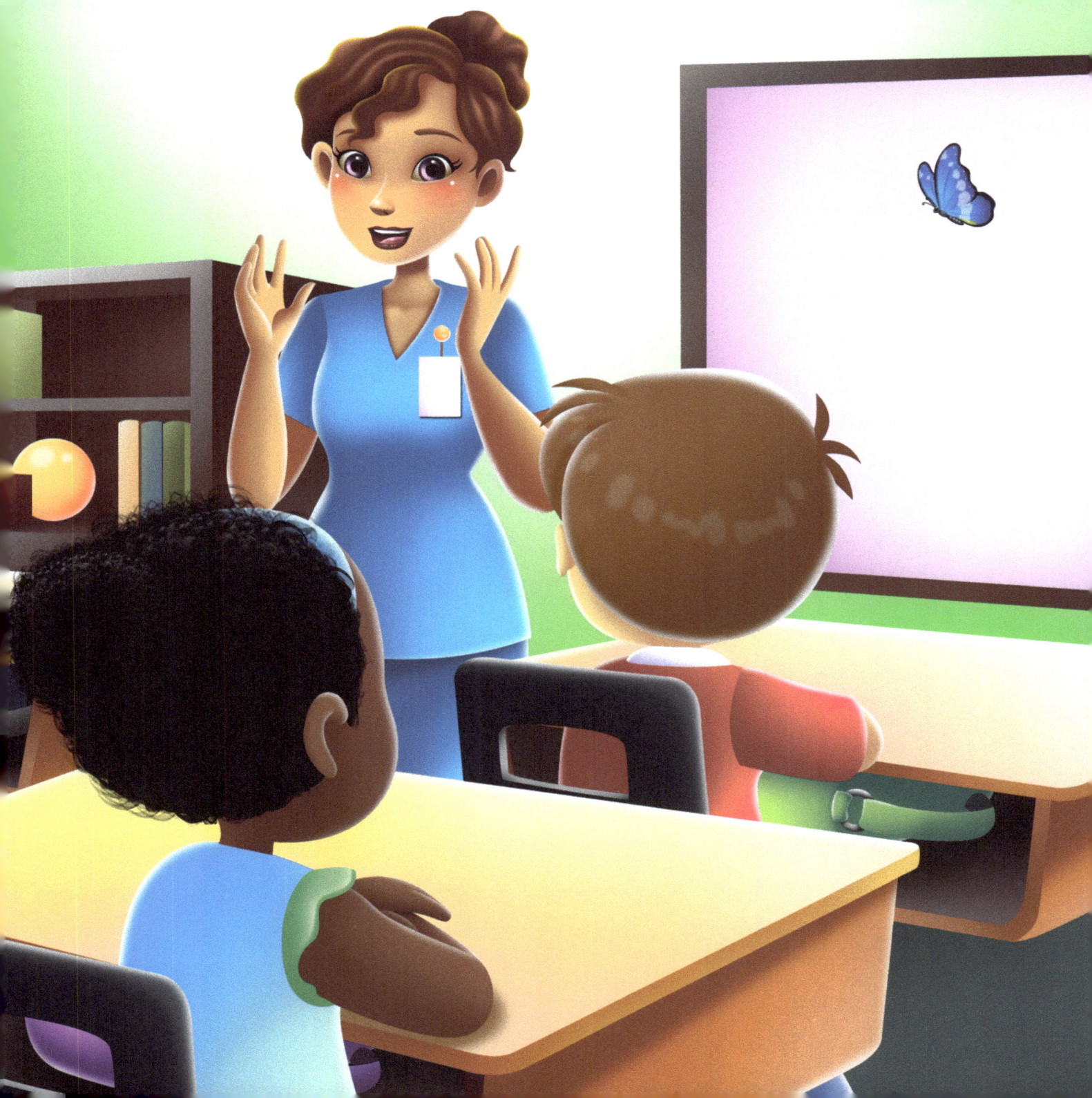

We learn we should wash our hands throughout the day, And talk about it again and again so we don't stray.

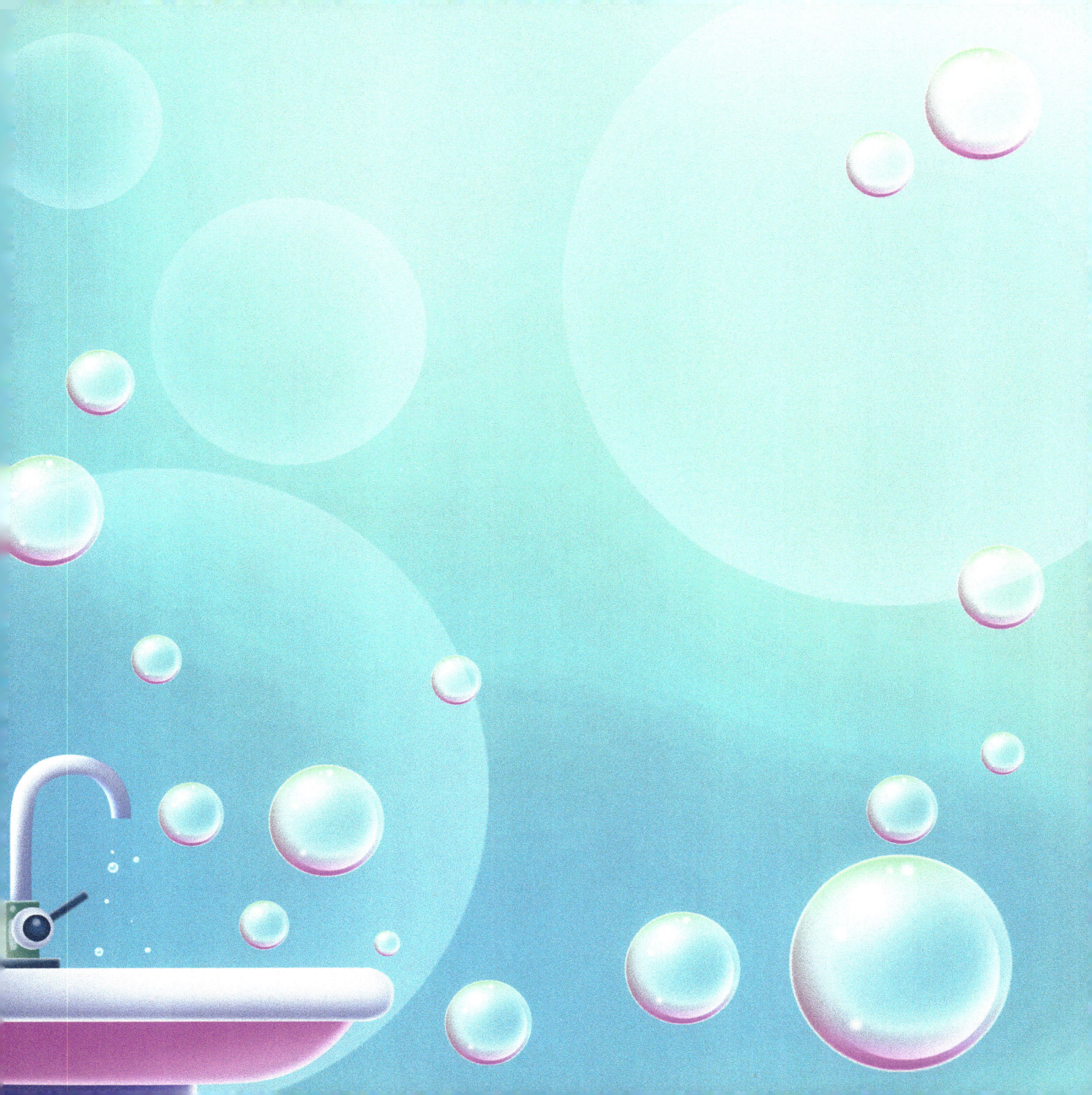

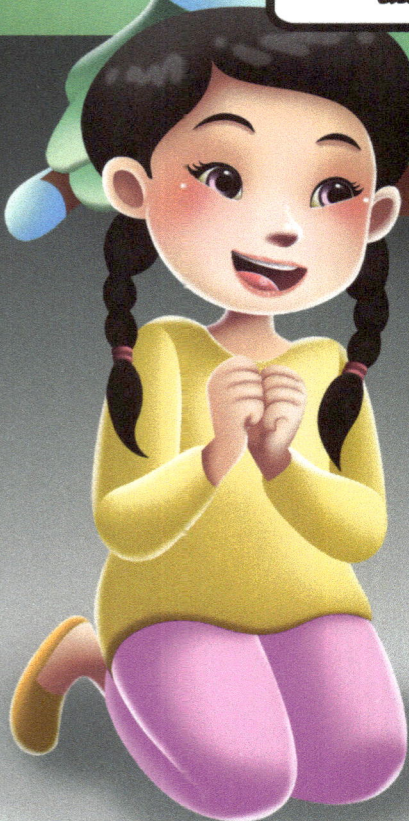

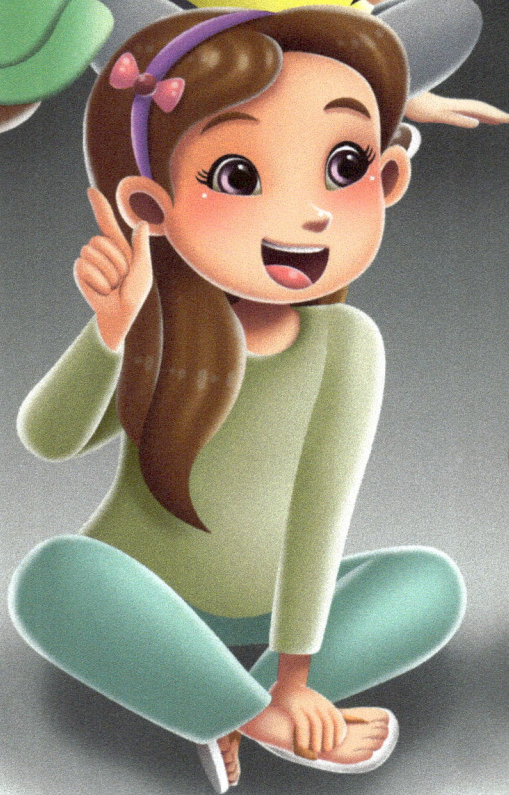

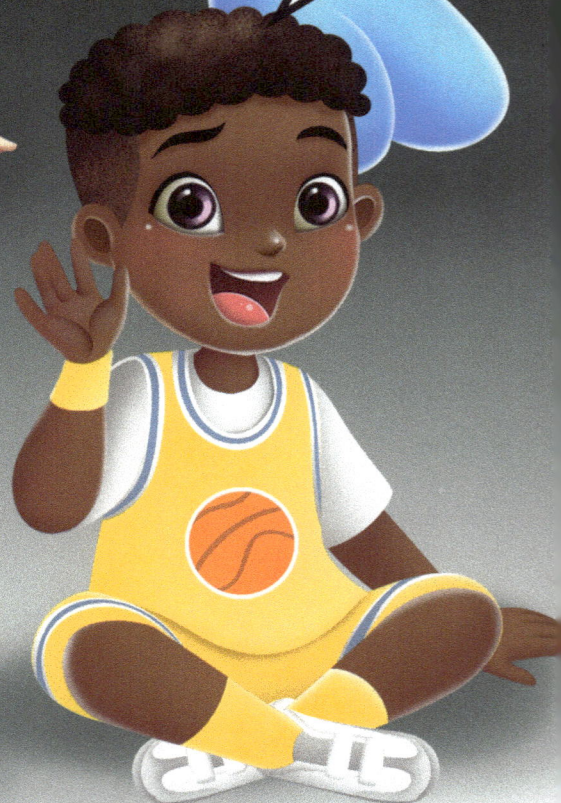

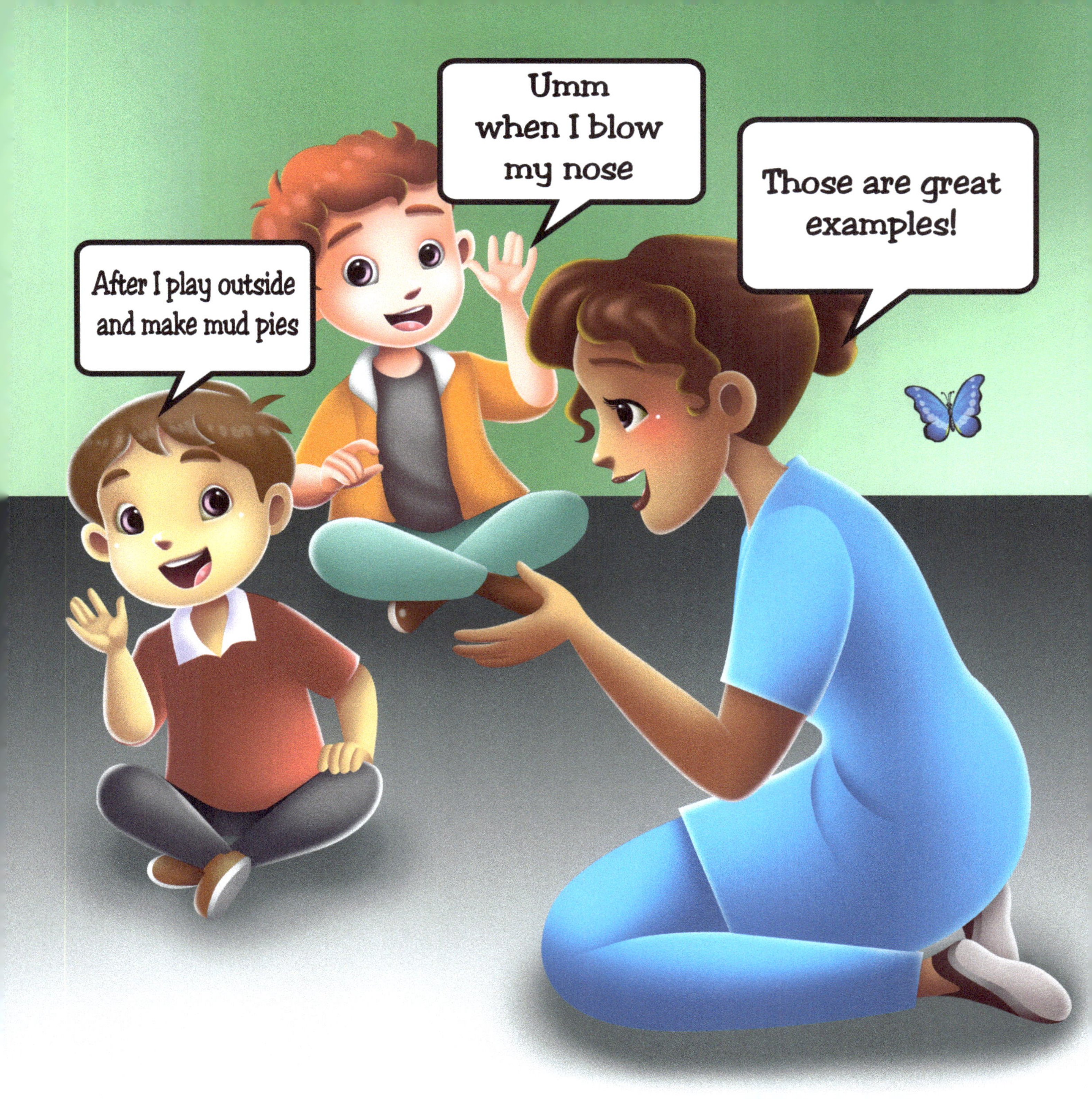
After I play outside and make mud pies
Umm when I blow my nose
Those are great examples!

We do not touch our nose, mouth, or eyelashes
Because we can spread those germs as quick as light
flashes. Washing our hands keeps others from getting sick.
I will say it again, washing your hands does the trick.

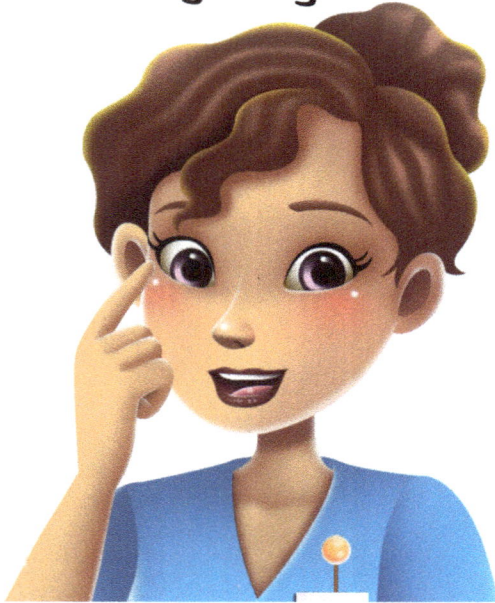

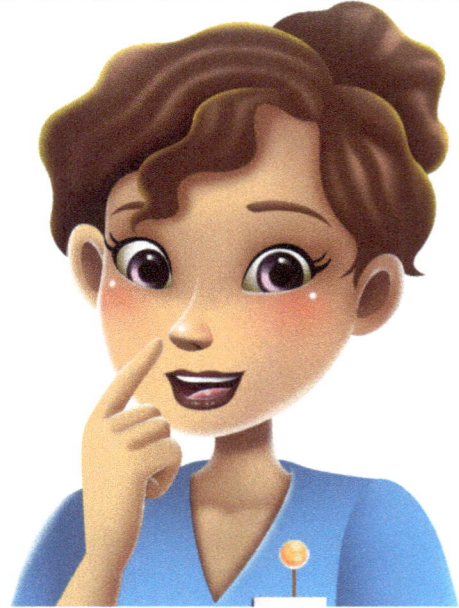

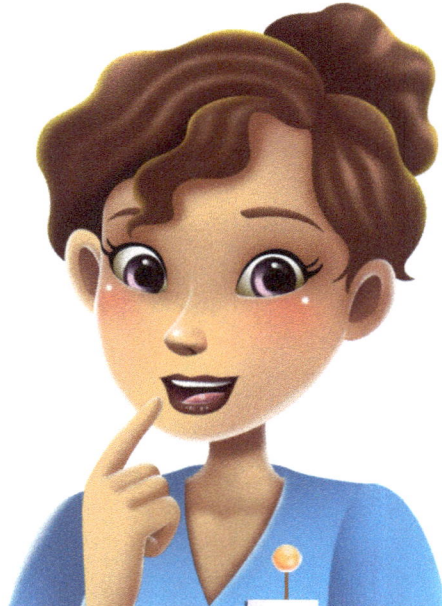

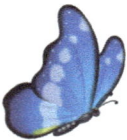

School was over, it was time to go home.
I see Baby Sis and zoom around her like
she is a stone. I have to wash my hands
before a hug and a kiss.

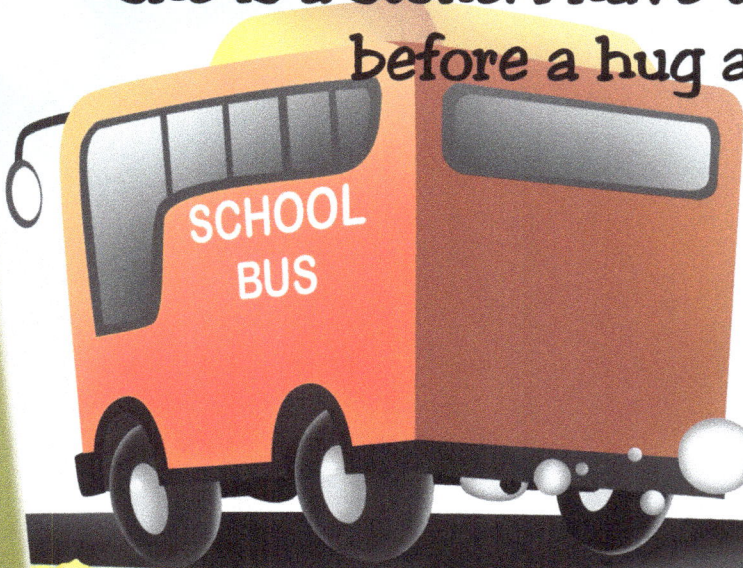

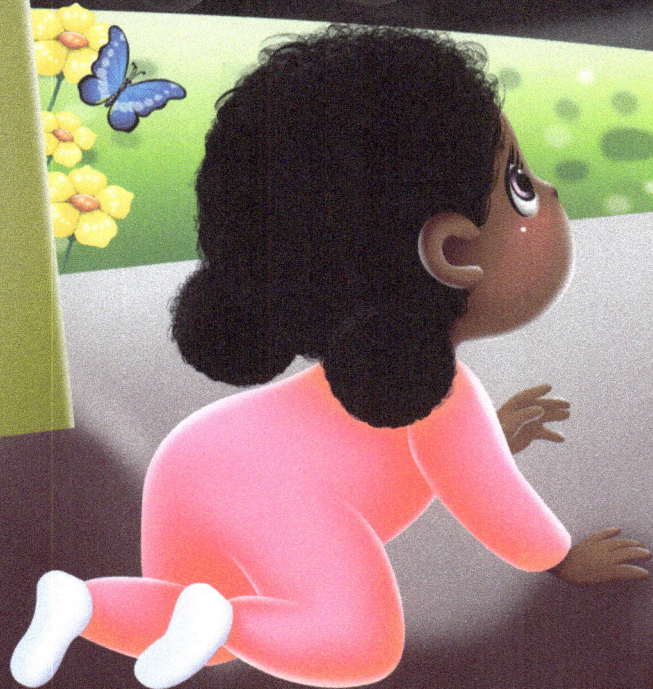

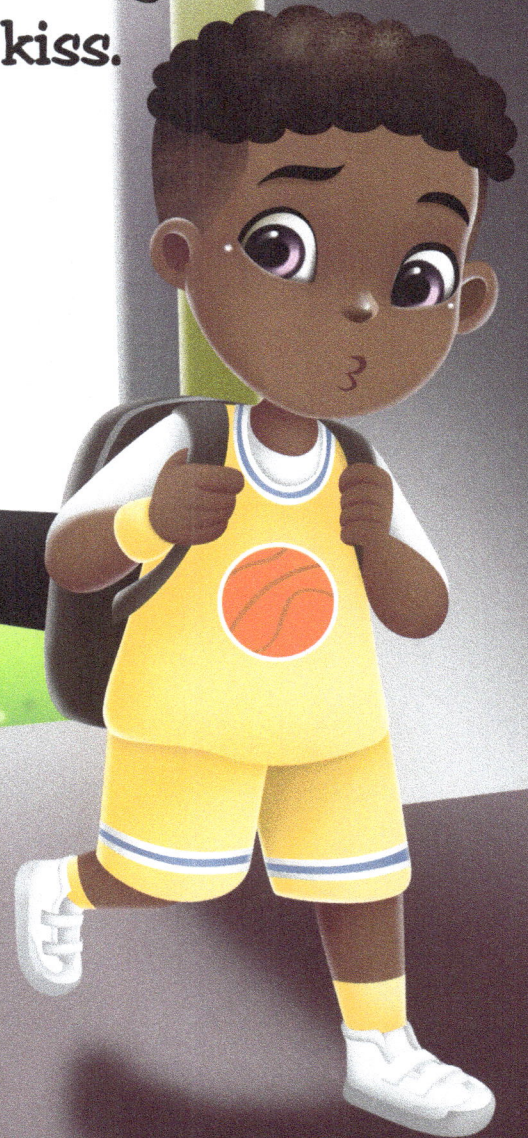

I motion to Baby Sis to come watch my hand washing show, I'm warming up my voice as she arrives at my elbow.

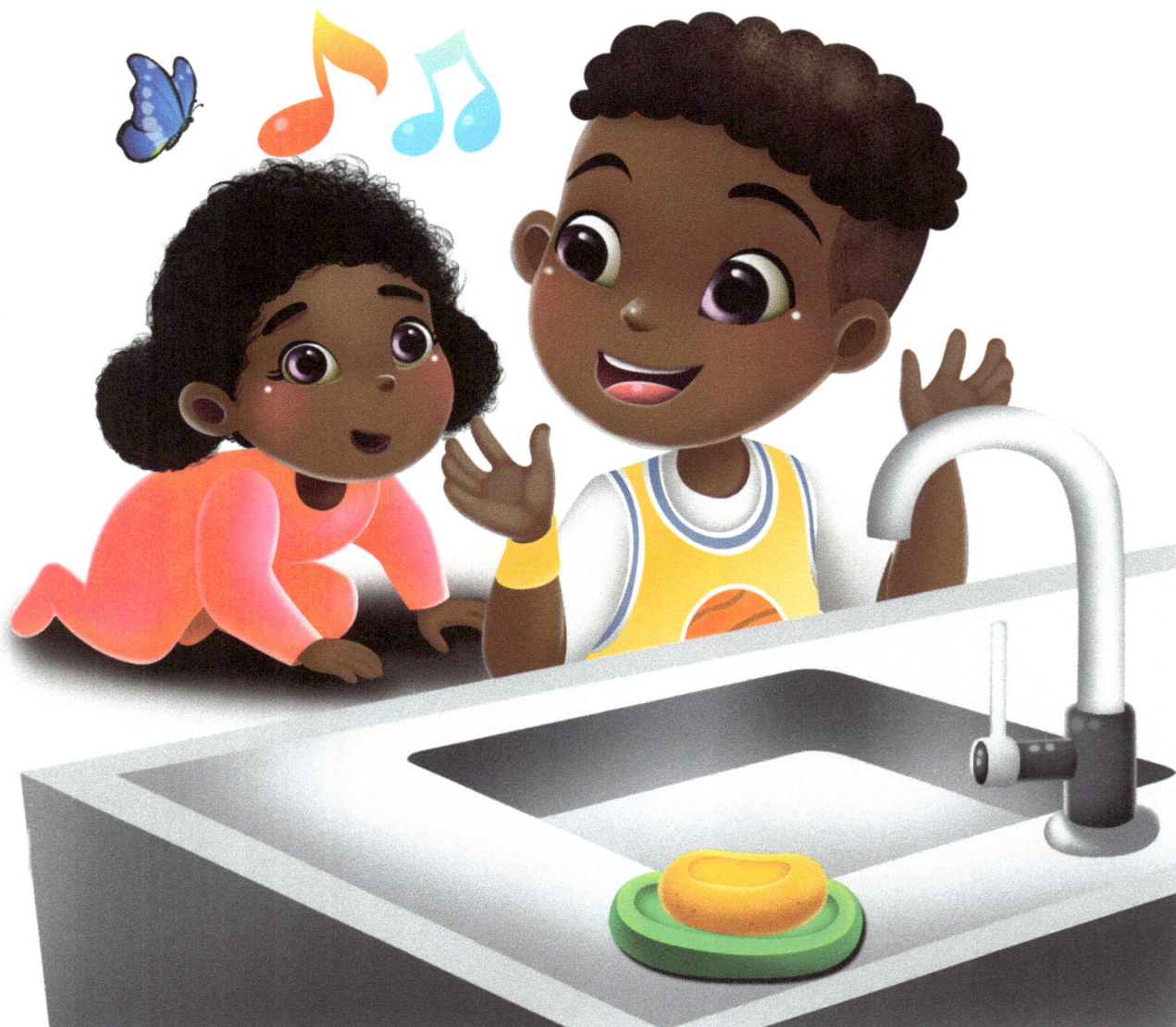

I go through the steps to show
her how it goes.

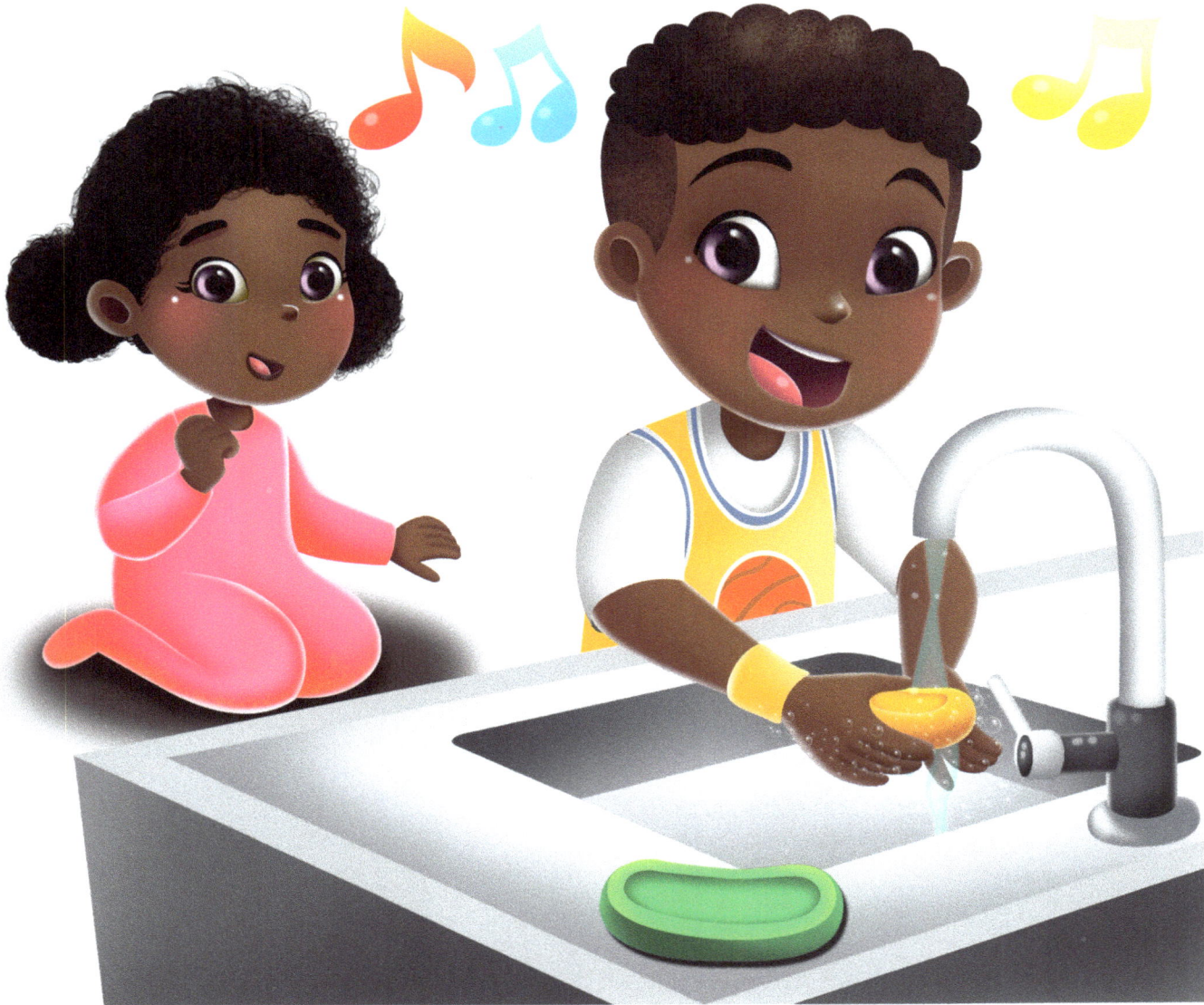

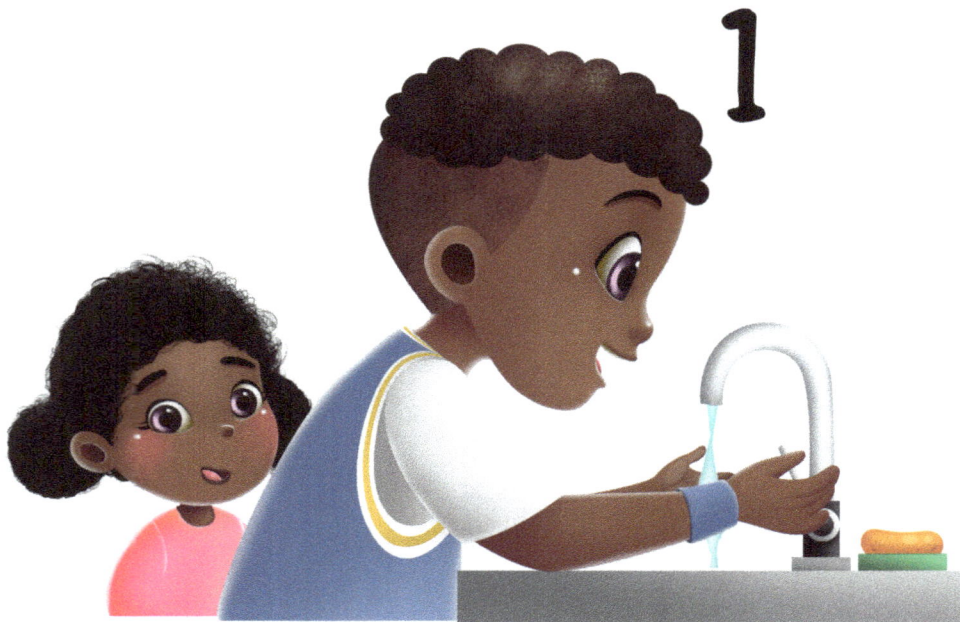

1

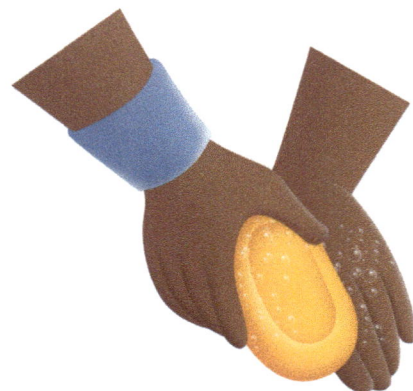

2

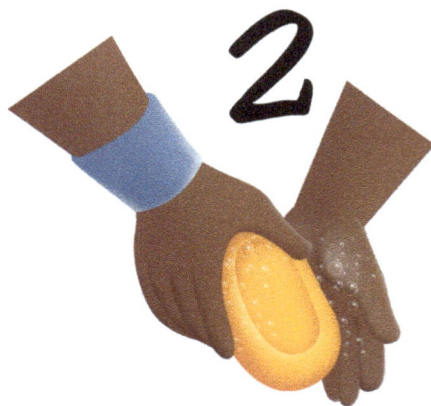

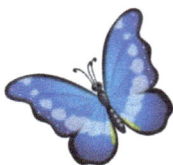

3

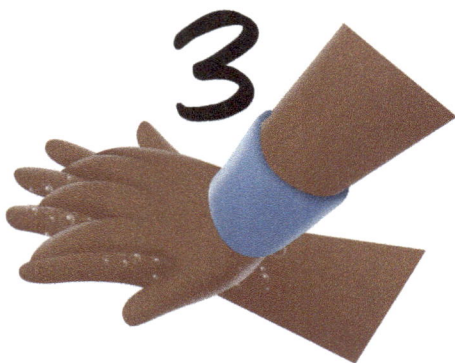

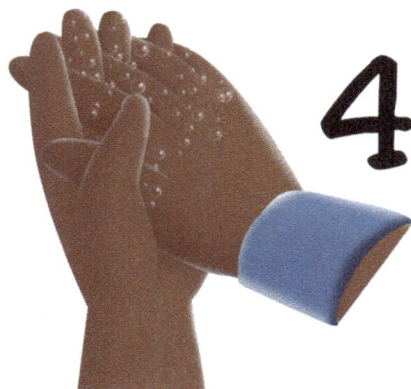

4

Step 1: Get your singing voice warmed
up "La, La, La."

Step 2: Turn the water on, rinse your
hands, and start singing the
Happy Birthday song.

Step 3: Rub soap on the front and back
of your hands and keep singing
your song.

Step 4: Wash in between and all around
each of your 10 fingers—start
with your thumb.

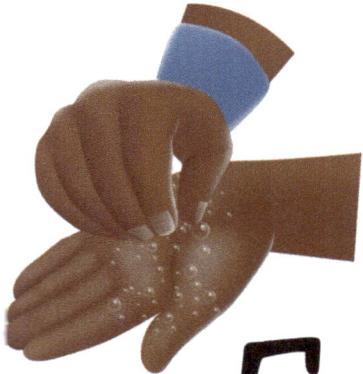

5

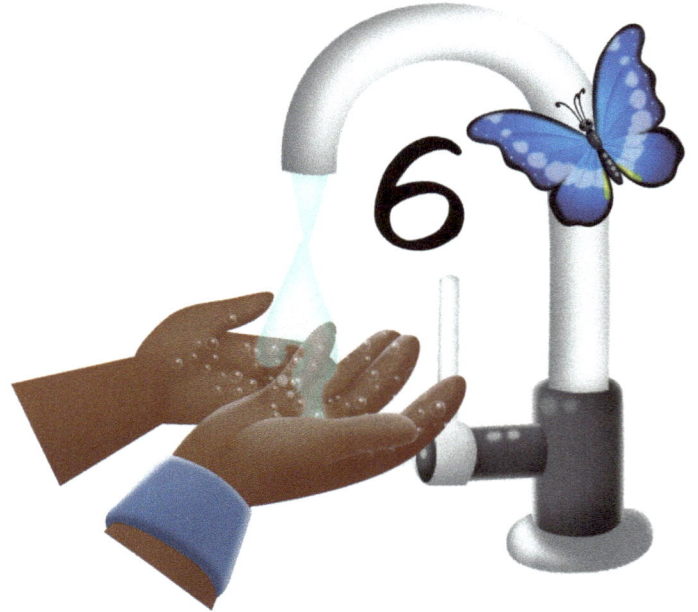

6

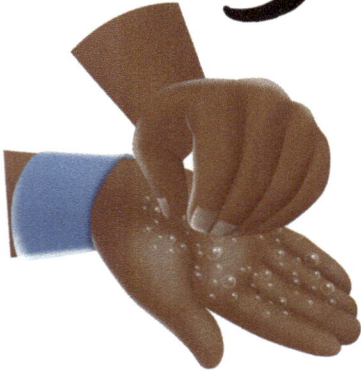

7

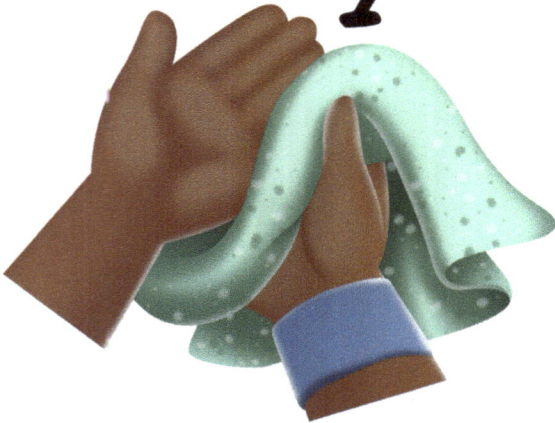

8

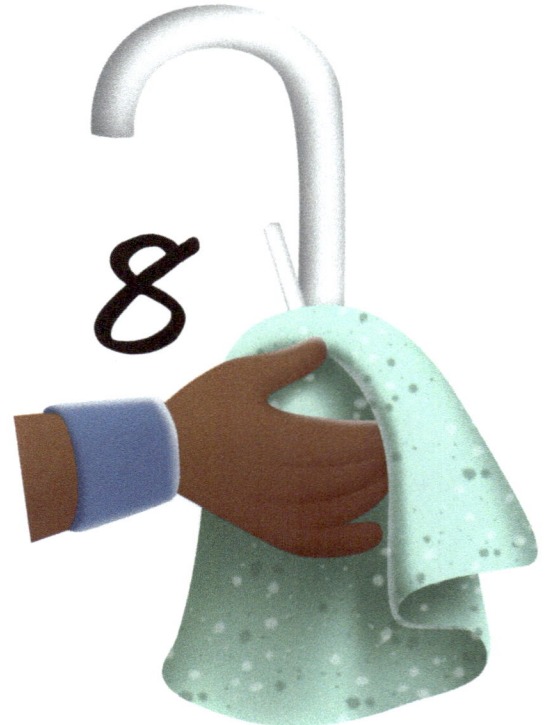

Step 5: Be sure to get underneath your fingernails while finishing up your song.

Step 6: Rinse all the soap off your hands with water.

Step 7: Dry your hands with a towel.

Step 8: Use that towel to turn off the faucet.

Baby Sis smiles and giggles as she is watching all this, I jump down and grab Baby Sis and give her a great big kiss.

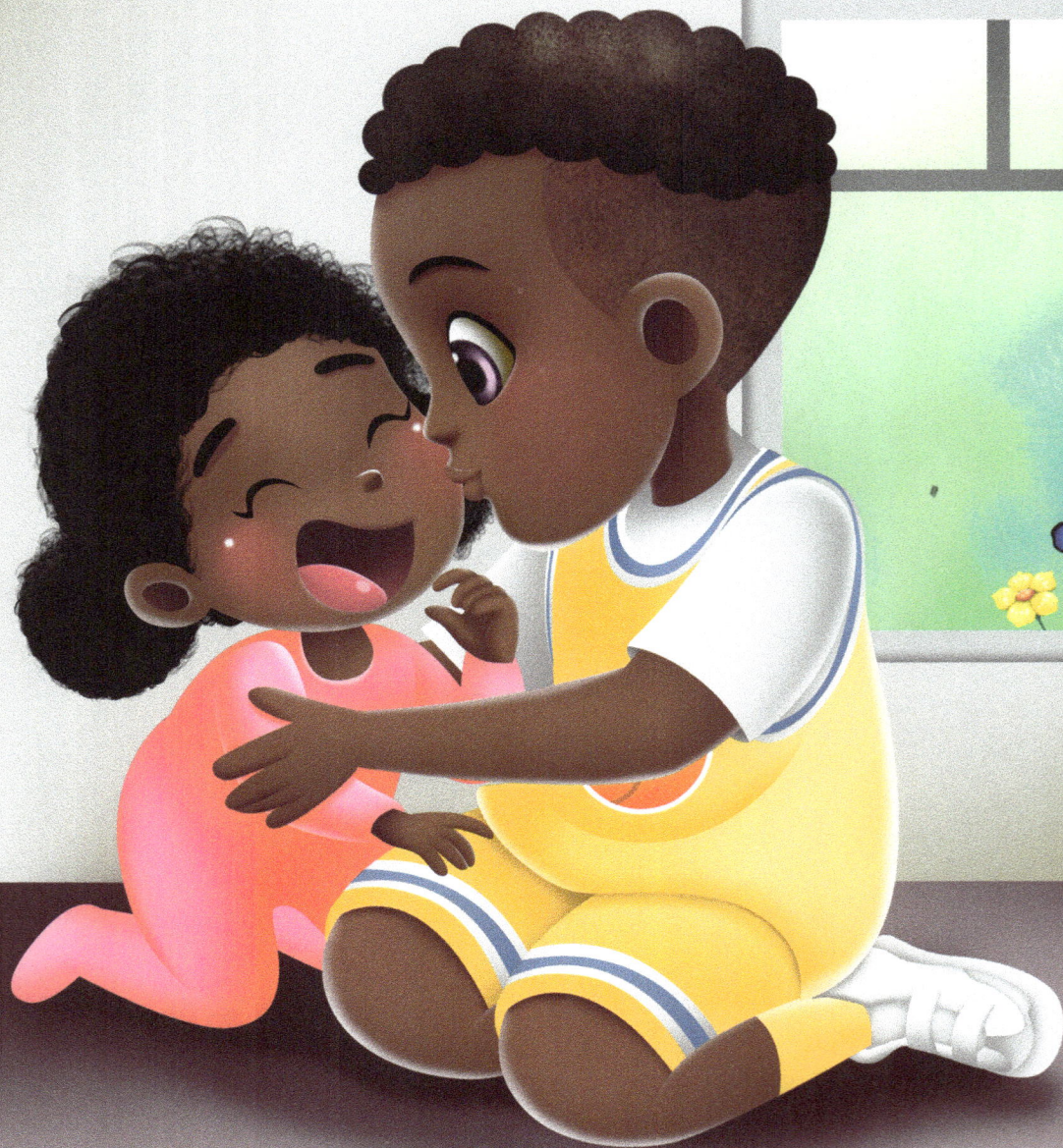

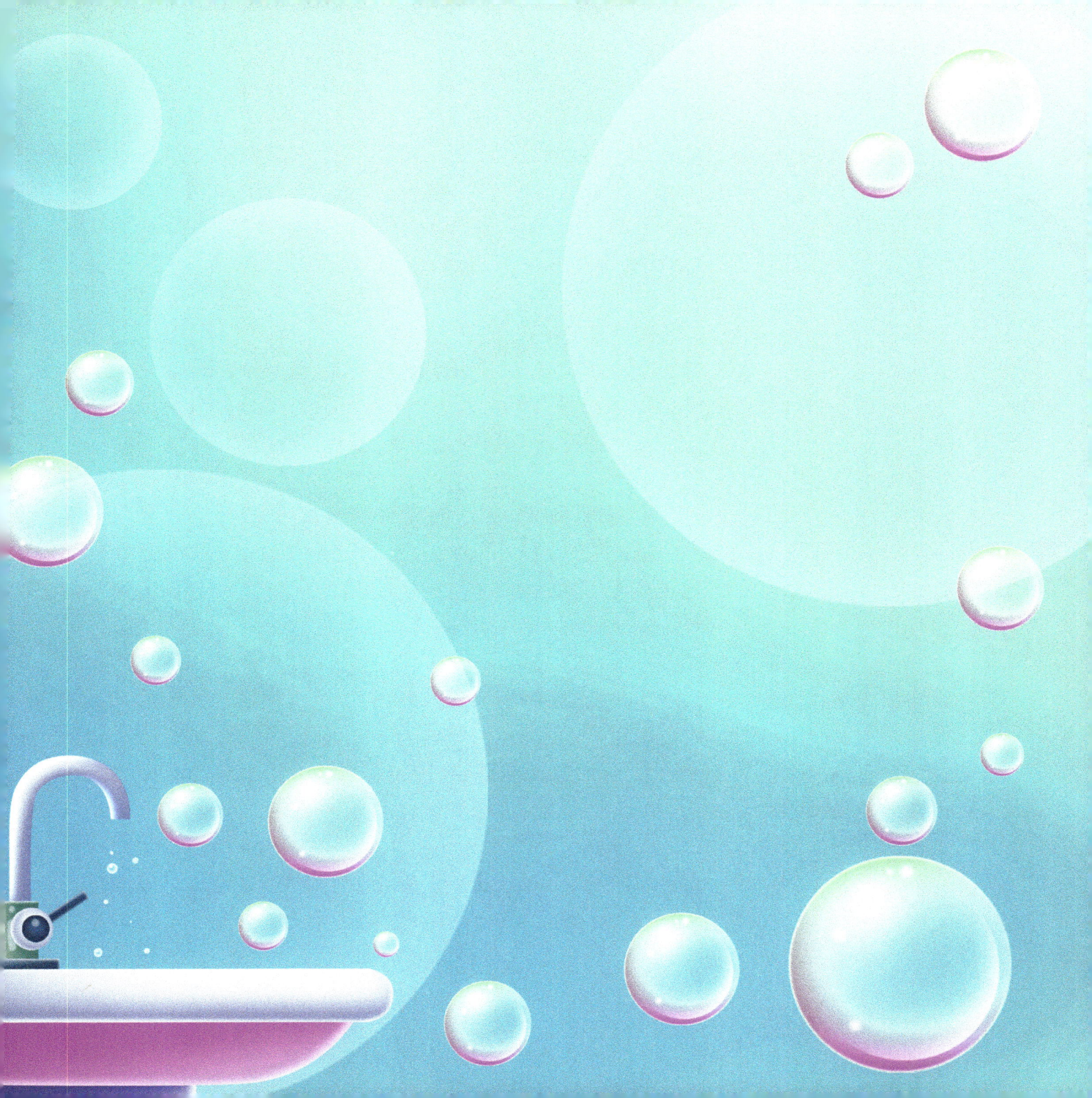

Hello Educators, Moms, Dads, and Loved ones!

Thank you for understanding the importance of teaching our kids the art of hand washing. If you didn't know, hand washing is our first line of defense to staying healthy. Washing hands helps stop the spread of germs and infecions.

As you read this story, show your kids how to wash their hands and then have them wash their own hands singing the Happy Birthday song. This song lasts about 15 seconds, the amount of time kids should wash their hands.

After washing hands, it is also important to not touch the sink faucet with your newly clean hands. Teach your kids to turn the faucet off with a paper towel or hand towel. The same goes for the bathroom door—use those paper or hand towels!

Ask your kids if they understand "when" and "why" they wash their hands. The questions Mrs. Tish asks in the story can help with this. If kids understand the "when" and "why" of hand washing, they will likely use the steps even when adults are not watching.

Thank you for all that you do in the life of a child. I hope this book helps you with the journey.

That's Love,
Erica

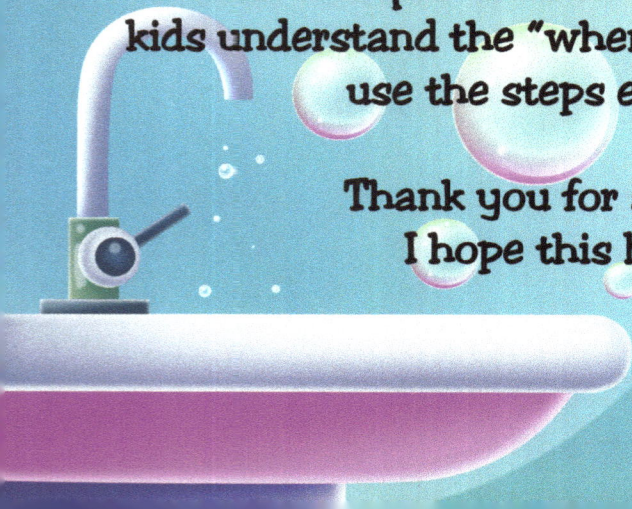

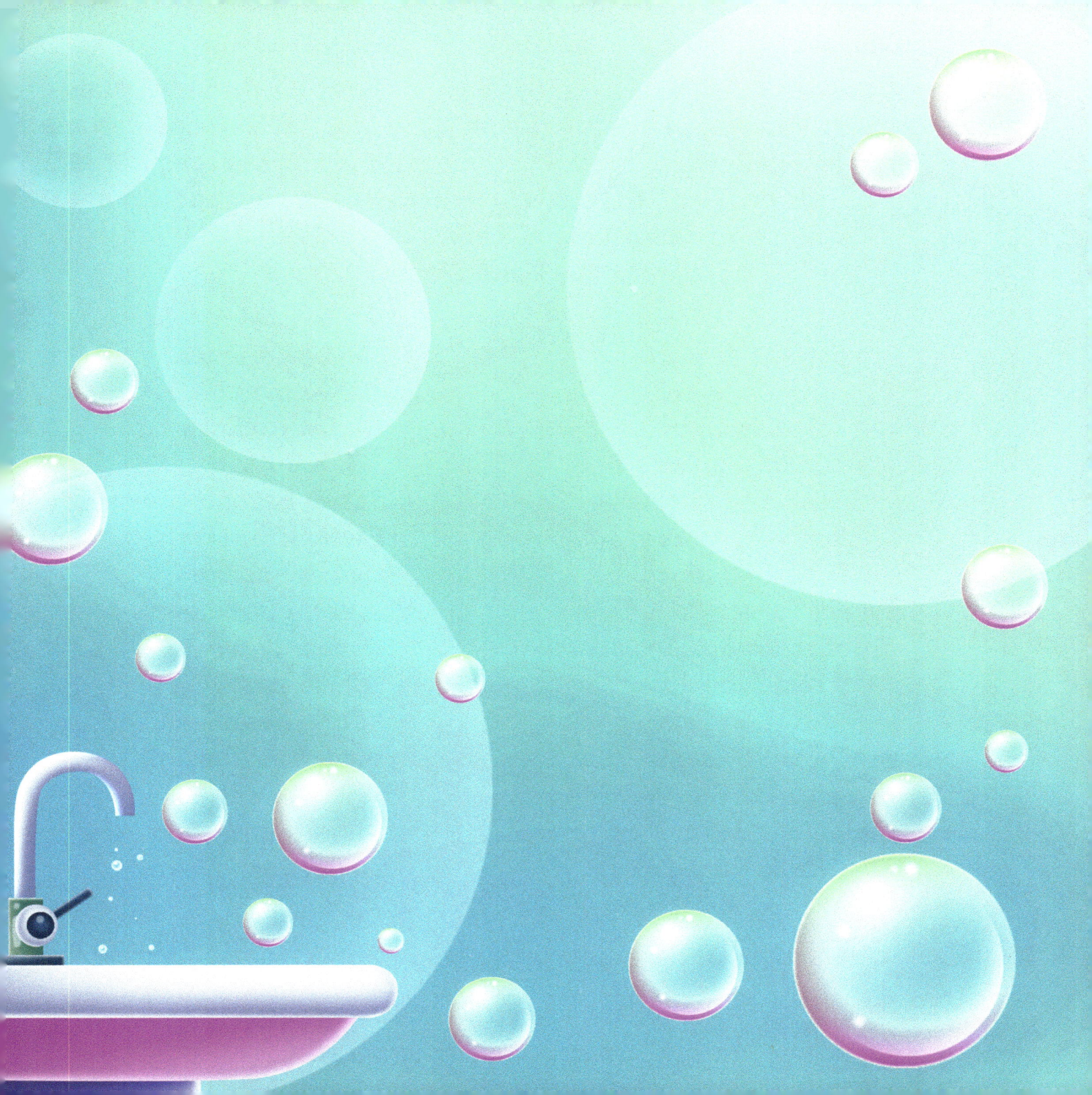

This page is dedicated to my Hand Washing Crew. All the individuals listed on this page played a role in helping the idea of this book become a reality. Each individual listed was encouraging and believed in the message of this book and the Little Miss series. Some even found my Kickstarter campaign page and supported there.
Thank you to the Hand Washing Crew.

Carmen Serrano
Ava Campbell
Jolyn Campbell
Eddie Basora
Claudia Nogueira
Anthony Moore
Pierre Jennings
Angela Turner Campbell
Robin Burnett Siesky
Lisa Pionzio
Laura Ramos
Pam Garcia
Shaunda Fennell
Jenni Wu
Erika James

Nydia Rodriguez
Lucretia Roman George
Shane Rollins
Gigi Sutton
Jacob Barnett
Emily Barnett
Ember Schake
Elsa Shay Carmody
Stephanie West
Sheri Pruett
Colin Evans
Dr. Chiamaka Agabasionwe
Zeide Arrosas
Juliana Alharahsheh
Jennie Cochran-Chinn

www.ingramcontent.com/pod-product-compliance
Lightning Source LLC
Chambersburg PA
CBHW042343030426
42335CB00030B/3443